The Politics of Youth, Sex, and Health Care in American Schools

T0315836

The Politics of Youth, Sex, and Health Care in American Schools

James W. Button, PhD
Barbara A. Rienzo, PhD

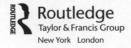

Routledge
Taylor & Francis Group
New York   London

First published 2002 by
The Haworth Press, Inc., 10 Alice Street, Binghamton, NY 13904-1580

This edition published 2013 by Routledge
711 Third Avenue, New York, NY 10017
2 Park Square, Milton Park, Abingdon, Oxon OX14 4RN

• • •• •••• • • •••• •• • ••• • •••• ••• •••• ••• • • ••• ••• •• •• ••• • ••• ••• •• • • ••• • •• • ••• • ••• •••

Cover design by Marylouise E. Doyle.

Library of Congress Cataloging-in-Publication Data

Button, James W., 1942-
    The politics of youth, sex, and health care in American schools / James W. Button, Barbara A. Rienzo.
        p. cm.
    Includes bibliographical references and index.
    ISBN 0-7890-1271-5 (alk. paper)—ISBN 0-7890-1272-3 (softcover : alk. paper)
    1. School health services—Political aspects—United States—Case studies. 2. Sex instruction for youth—Political aspects—United States—Case studies. I. Rienzo, Barbara Ann. II. Title.

LB3409.U5 B88 2002
371.7'1—dc21

                                         2002068771

CONTENTS

ABOUT THE AUTHORS

James W. Button, PhD, is Professor of Political Science at the University of Florida in Gainesville. He specializes in the study of local politics, including the politics of education, minority politics, and the processes of social change. He has numerous scholarly publications to his name, including the V. O. Key Book Award–winning *Blacks and Social Change: The Impact of the Civil Rights Movement in Southern Communities*. He has been awarded a number of grants to explore race, politics, and community change.

Barbara A. Rienzo, PhD, is Professor of Health Science Education at the University of Florida in Gainesville. Her expertise is in the areas of human sexuality and health education. She has published numerous scholarly articles and book chapters and has consulted extensively with school districts nationally on teacher training and sexuality education program implementation. She has been awarded some $420,000 in grant funds that have supported both research and the development of health promotion materials for schools. She was one of 30 initial recipients of University of Florida Research Professorship Awards (1997-2000).

Preface

"Seesaw Battle Goes on Over School Clinic in Gadsden"; "Neighborhood Clinic Praised; Teenage Pregnancies Reduced by Approximately 75 Percent"; "Clinic Is Moved Back to Campus After Three Years Across the Street"—such were the headlines in north Florida newspapers that grabbed our attention more than ten years ago and precipitated this study. With the authors' expertise in human sexuality education (BR) and politics of social change (JB), we were uniquely prepared to attend to the question: what are the crucial political factors that affect controversial yet successful public health programs such as school-based health clinics? We knew, for example, that almost 11 million children (one in six) lacked medical insurance, and millions more were uninsured for parts of the year. School-based health centers (SBHCs) began as an innovative grassroots effort to fill this void in the nation's health care delivery system. Another basic goal of SBHCs was to address issues of reproductive health care, particularly the high rates of teenage pregnancy and sexually transmitted diseases. Moreover, children in poverty (approximately 20 percent of American youths) have greater and more frequent health problems that in turn have a notable impact on their school performance. SBHCs contribute directly to improving the academic achievement and social behavior of students by ameliorating some of the causes of poor performance. Thus we embarked upon what turned out to be a decade-long look at the political process that influences the establishment, growth, and ultimate success of this important education and health care innovation.

Our intent in writing this book is threefold. First, we want to make information relevant to the politics of health accessible to those dedicated medical, education, and social service professionals in the field. All too often the crucial skills involved in building support and dealing with resistance (i.e., "politics") are missing from professional preparation. As a result, promising programs are not often given a chance to succeed due to the inability of schools and communities to get beyond initial hurdles. Second, we hope this study contributes to the body of knowledge that scholars of school and health politics need to optimize chances for implementing innovation to improve the health of youth (and their families). School health centers have often encountered substantial political resistance, and scholars have considered the emerging conflicts as one example of current culture war issues confronting schools. Third and last, we hope that our research contributes to the public's vision of the possible—that important changes can be instituted through "politics" as usual. This study analyzes not only the nature and extent of political barriers but, more important, what strategies have proved most successful in overcoming these barriers.

Some of the more technical aspects of this study have been reported in scholarly journal articles. Thus scholars and students can access the specific research findings and analyses in those sources (cited throughout this book). The information presented herein focuses mainly on the details regarding how and why innovations such as school health centers occur and continue. We have deliberately limited tables, figures, and statistics. Instead, we include descriptions of the people and the methods they used and whenever possible use their words to give voice to the important lessons learned.

This study is unique not only in that the political process underlying the effective implementation of an important school health innovation is revealed but also because it presents information on how programs maintain and grow over time. We began our investigation in 1991-1992 and revisited school-based clinics in 1998-1999. At both junctures, two types of research methods were utilized: we employed a national survey that provided the overall picture in time and the quantitative data necessary to explore contextual factors; and we conducted case studies of five representative school communities, which provided a rich source of qualitative information that described and explained basic findings.

We are very grateful to the Spencer Foundation (Chicago), a national organization that supports research on programs in education, and to the University of Florida Division of Sponsored Research for funding this study. We also express our utmost appreciation to the variety of respondents considered knowledgeable about clinic evolution and politics in each community whom we interviewed in both the early and late 1990s. Those interviewed typically included clinic coordinators and staff, school administrators, teachers, parents, school board members, leaders of community and political groups both supportive and in opposition to clinics, and media representatives. Local newspapers and available clinic records added further depth. The research assistance we received from our students, especially Seth McKee, was crucial. To our colleague and good friend, Ken Wald, goes our utmost regard and appreciation. Ken's insights, especially related to research design and his contributions to the research analysis, were invaluable.

Finally, we must acknowledge with deepest gratitude the contributions of our families and friends. They are our abiding supporters and our loyal readership. They form our sacred circle.

Chapter 1

Evolution of Health Services in Schools

Angela is an 18-year-old Hispanic high school student in Prince George's County, Maryland, who suffers from asthma, disabling migraines, and worries about getting pregnant. She comes from a poor family that she has left, works two jobs to support herself, and has no health insurance.

Washington Post, February 1, 1994

Sam, an eleventh-grade African-American student in Jersey City, New Jersey, lost his mother last year and faces so many problems at home that he almost left. He's very depressed; he has no easy access to condoms, and he thinks that his girlfriend may be pregnant and that he has an STD.

Interview, May 19, 1999

In the last several decades youth in American society have undergone dramatic changes. Among all age groups, children and adolescents now have the highest rates of poverty. Today 25 percent of youth live in families with only one parent, more than double the rate of two decades ago. More than 50 percent of these single-parent children live in poverty. For growing numbers of African-American and Hispanic youth, all of these figures depicting rates of poverty and social and economic disadvantage are much higher. Amid the deteriorating conditions for youth, health care and housing costs have increased significantly. At the same time, budget crises and anti-government rhetoric at all levels have produced drastic cuts in health and social services. These contending forces—the increased needs of children and deep concerns over public spending—have exacerbated a serious crisis for many of America's youth. All of this has contributed to the explosion of the "new morbidities"—unprotected sexual behavior, substance abuse, depression, and violence—that continually threaten the well-being of today's children and tomorrow's adults.

At the community and school level, a number of innovative approaches have been discussed and a few implemented to confront this growing crisis. One of the most unique and successful interventions has combined health and social services within educational institutions in what are called school-based health centers (SBHCs). Beginning almost three decades ago, community health agencies and schools in Dallas, Texas, and St. Paul, Minnesota, implemented plans to provide health care to underserved youth through their schools, especially services to combat high teen pregnancy rates. This partnership between health and education seemed an inexpensive and expedient way to meet the pressing physical and social problems affecting students in low-income families. School-based health centers proved to be so successful that today more than 1,000 communities across the country have adopted this school and health care reform in one or more of their schools—a reform that now involves national and local foundations, every level of government, health care institutions, universities, and many professional organizations. From serving poor and minority youth, SBHCs increasingly have grown to provide health services to children and teens in more middle-class neighborhoods.

Our primary goal is to reveal the history, nature, and political dynamics involved in building and sustaining this important innovation in delivering health and social care to youth and, increasingly, their families. Clearly it is important to understand why and how SBHCs began and how they have persisted amid budget concerns, growing health care demands, and frequent criticisms of the schools. Despite their dramatic increase in numbers, SBHCs have nonetheless confronted a number of issues that have ultimately limited the development and growth of this unique program of health care. Among the most important barriers have been consistent and continuous funding, lack of full parental and community support, misunderstanding and poor communication between health professionals and educators, conflicts with some physicians in the community and with school nurses, and, most significant, the politically controversial nature of some services, especially the provision of reproductive health care for teens. Because of these highly controversial services, clinics have often encountered substantial political resistance, and many observers have considered the emerging conflicts as one example of current culture war issues confronting U.S. schools. These and other political conflicts have limited the growth and funding of SBHCs. We shall not only analyze the nature and extent of such political issues and controversies but also discuss what strategies have proved most successful in overcoming these barriers. Since the American educational system is decentralized, initiating and sustaining such reform involves building local support and overcoming the opposition. This is the "politics" of school-based health care, or of any school innovation, and it is an essential but often neglected aspect of reform.

HEALTH STATUS AND CARE
OF AMERICAN YOUTH

Access to health care is a significant issue for America's youth. This is largely due to the fact that the poverty rate for those under age eighteen (approximately 20 percent) is much higher than for the rest of the population. Living in poverty is also a function of race and ethnicity, with almost 40 percent of African-American and Hispanic youth in this category. About 12 million American youth are medically uninsured and millions of others have inadequate insurance that fails, for example, to cover even basic immunizations necessary for school attendance. Studies also show that schools with poorer students report high rates of unsafe school environments, another significant health risk for these children. Finally, according to a 1997 Institute of Medicine report (Eng and Butler, 1997), even adolescents with access to care rarely get help for problems of greatest importance, because most physicians are untrained and feel unqualified to address these issues. Those with mental health and dental problems, which comprise a significant number of youth, go largely untreated (Allensworth et al., 1997).

Youth in lower socioeconomic levels suffer disproportionate rates of all types of risks associated with morbidity and mortality. In the 1980s it was found that these risk behaviors (substance abuse, sexual activity, delinquency, depression, and school problems) were interrelated and that approximately 25 percent of America's youth were at high risk for the problems that resulted from these behaviors. Today the estimated numbers of youth who are at "high risk" or "very high risk" have increased to approximately 35 percent (Dryfoos, 1998).

Youth sexual behavior, in particular, has caused professionals to create school-based programs to help adolescents avoid the plethora of problems resulting from unintended pregnancies and sexually transmitted diseases. Almost 80 percent of males and 66 percent of females initiated sexual intercourse during their teenage years. Studies also have shown that teens wait at least a year or more after initiating intercourse before acquiring a medical form of contraception. More than 1 million teenage females become pregnant each year. Four in ten become pregnant at least once before age twenty. Of these, about 40 percent of pregnancies are terminated through elective abortion, and nearly 500,000 infants are born to mothers age nineteen or younger. Most teens do not use condoms at all or use them inconsistently. Thus, their vulnerability to sexually transmitted diseases, including HIV, also becomes a cause of concern. Adolescents account for at least 25 percent of the more than 15 million cases of STDs that occur annually in the United States. Moreover, STDs among adolescents are causally related to HIV, infertility, cervical cancers, spontaneous abortion, and low-birth-weight infants (Bar-Cohen, Lia-Hoagberg, and Edwards, 1990; Crosby and Lawrence, 2000).

SCHOOLS AND HEALTH CARE

Health problems suffered by these youth are clearly related to difficulties in learning and poor school achievement. Recognizing this, the American Academy of Pediatrics has supported comprehensive school health programs due to the conviction that such interventions increase the "health and educational outcomes of youth" (1993:4). The "comprehensive school health program," a concept introduced in the 1980s, includes a broad range of school-based and community-based activities all designed to prevent disease, promote health, and minimize the complications of health problems of school-age children. Of the seven primary goals of comprehensive school health programs, four involve school-based medical care services and personnel: assuring access to primary care, providing a system for dealing with medical crises, providing medical screening and immunizations, and identifying and resolving students' health and educational problems. In addition to medical care, school services that are part of this model include health education, healthful environment, health promotion, physical education, nutrition, and mental health counseling. Unfortunately, very few schools have implemented a truly comprehensive school health program.

Nonetheless, schools have been central in efforts to provide a wide range of health and social services for American children since the inception of compulsory education in the mid-1800s. At the turn of the nineteenth century, schools in large urban areas were used to deliver health and social services to children, particularly those children of immigrants. Controlling smallpox and other communicable diseases was a major concern among medical and public health officials, and schools were recognized as the logical place of access to children. Medical "inspections" of youth in schools by health personnel were initiated in Boston, New York, Philadelphia, Chicago, and other major cities. School nurses soon assumed the role of inspecting students, treating minor ailments at school, and referring major problems to physicians. Yet the number of schools that had nurses or medical personnel was few, and the focus was limited to youth with recognized needs (Means, 1975).

World War I had a decided impact on school health programs. The poor physical condition of many war draftees, especially those living in poverty, led to a greater emphasis on health care for youth. Immediately after the war, almost all states enacted legislation calling for health and physical education for schoolchildren. Yet schools were reluctant to provide comprehensive health services. School nurses, or sometimes nurses' aides, focused on first aid, health screenings, and preventive health care. It was assumed that most youth had family doctors for primary care, and the appropriate role of schools was to inform parents of health problems or refer students to community health services (Allensworth et al., 1997; Kort, 1984).

The advent of the War on Poverty and Great Society programs of the 1960s marked another watershed for education and health care. Federal legislation established Head Start, Medicaid, free or reduced school lunch programs, and Title I of the Elementary and Secondary Education Act of 1965, all of which provided new funds for and emphasis on school health and social services. Recognizing and meeting the needs of poverty-ridden students was a primary concern. As a result, health and school officials became more aware of the issues of drug abuse, teen pregnancy, sexually transmitted diseases, emotional health, and malnutrition that affected significant numbers of children and adolescents. With the influx of public funding for schools and health care, a number of programs were instituted that focused on the potential for schools to meet the special needs of the young.

Another factor that influenced the development and focus of health care was the black civil rights movement in the 1960s. The focus of this movement was on equal rights for African Americans, and these rights included health care and education. The mass mobilization and protests of blacks, first in the South and later in the urban ghettos of the North, highlighted the poverty and social disadvantages of African-American youth as well as adults. Compared to white youth, black children were much more likely to live in a single-parent household, often with an adolescent mother, and to have parents who had not completed high school. Almost half of all African-American youth lived in poverty (Jaynes and Williams, 1989). The black movement, and somewhat later the Hispanic movement, focused greater attention on the morbidities of black and Latino youth, and education and health professionals sought more government funding and new approaches to deal with what had been an "invisible" minority population. Thus, events of the 1960s elevated issues of race, ethnicity, and poverty, including their effects on youth, to the national political agenda.

More recently, pressures have been mounting for schools to expand health care for youth, particularly due to the realization that certain health behaviors are responsible for 70 percent of adolescent mortality and morbidity. According to the Centers for Disease Control and Prevention, these health behaviors include unintentional and intentional injuries, drug and alcohol abuse, sexually transmitted diseases and unintended pregnancies, diseases associated with tobacco use, illnesses resulting from inadequate physical activity, mental disorders, and problems due to inadequate dietary patterns (Allensworth et al., 1997). Along with the recognition of the growing need for services, especially among poorer youth, has been the understanding that schools are the primary venue where children may be reached.

A further impetus for providing health care for youth was the National Education Goals initiative, which originated at a national governors' summit in 1989, and emphasized that students begin school with the health status necessary for learning. Goals of these bipartisan guidelines stressed school health and stated that schools should provide safe environments that are free of drugs and alcohol, and that school districts should implement health and physical education classes. Another significant influence on schools was the U.S. Public Health Service initiative Healthy People 2000: of the almost 300 objectives for health promotion and disease prevention for the nation, one-third were identified as achievable in part or wholly through the schools (Allensworth et al., 1997). By 1995, the majority of schools offered some form of prevention programming. Although not all such programs have been developed well or proven very effective, most school districts have some curricula to prevent smoking, alcohol use, and drug use, can screen for physical health problems, and have some form of sexuality education (Durlak, 1995).

THE DEVELOPMENT OF SCHOOL-BASED CLINICS

Clearly a consensus is growing among educational reformers and child and youth advocates: schools must increase their capacity for providing a wide range of health, social, and other services to meet the growing needs of at-risk students. This is an admission that traditionally structured schools cannot begin to solve the complex social, economic, and family problems that affect many youth. School nurses are not able to care for all the injuries; guidance counselors cannot deal with the rising incidence of depression and violence; and other school personnel do not have the time or training to cope with the "new morbidities." It has become increasingly apparent that the American educational system was not developed to address twenty-first-century issues of sexuality, drugs, violence, and homelessness (Dryfoos, 1991).

The focus on schools as providers of comprehensive health care has resulted from recognition that school performance is greatly affected by the social, economic, and physical problems of youth. This is especially the case for children and adolescents who come from poor and disadvantaged families. These young people often suffer from poor health, physical disabilities, and malnutrition as well. Moreover, such high-risk youth are the least likely to have access to health care. These behaviors and conditions clearly have a major impact on school performance.

With conventional school health care consisting of a school nurse (or less), there has been a growing demand for substantial interventions in and out of schools to try to change the behaviors and improve the living conditions of at-risk students. Teachers and other school staff are situated to identify early-on emerging social or health problems. Thus the idea to locate comprehensive medical clinics within schools was an appealing one because SBHCs offer easy access to health services by bringing providers to youth. Typically furnishing free or low-cost services within an atmosphere of trust and confidentiality, school-based health centers provide a continuity of care not available elsewhere for many youth.

School health clinics are a relatively new idea. The first roots of a center took hold in 1967 in Cambridge (MA) when a pediatrician, head of child health for the city health department, hired a nurse practitioner to establish a clinic in an elementary school rather than in the health department. Providing medical services at school seemed a more efficient way to meet the health needs of children. Two years later SBHCs were opened in two elementary schools in West Dallas (TX) with federal funding that was part of the War on Poverty. In the same city, the first center to offer comprehensive services in a high school was begun in 1970 as an outreach project of the University of Texas Health Sciences Center. "We started our clinics in elementary schools first because that's where the highest rates of morbidity and mortality were occurring among poor children," claimed the manager of the West Dallas centers. "We expanded our services into the high school almost immediately because we noticed that there was a tremendous need for service in adolescents as well" (Making the Grade, 1998:1).

High teen pregnancy rates provided the impetus for the beginnings of several centers in the 1970s. In 1973 in St. Paul (MN), for example, the Maternal-Infant Care Program at a medical center started a high school clinic to serve pregnant and parenting teens. One of the rationales for the West Dallas High School (TX) health center also had been to provide family planning services that were unavailable to youth in the community. In St. Paul, the program was initiated by an obstetrician who had observed directly the problems related to high rates of teen pregnancy and childbirth. Plagued by low enrollments, the clinic expanded to include comprehensive health services, and the numbers of clients climbed. Early reports of the clinic's success in reducing childbearing created considerable publicity and stimulated consideration of SBHCs as a new approach to adolescent pregnancy prevention (Dryfoos, 1994). Reported birthrates in St. Paul high schools with clinics declined from fifty-nine births per 1,000 female students in 1976-1977 to twenty-six per 1,000 in 1983-1984. The program was also attributed with reducing teens' abortion rates due to a decline in the number of pregnancies. In addition, these clinics served a high proportion of teenage females for family planning needs, increased their continuation rates of effective contraception use within sexual relationships, and kept parenting mothers in school (Dryfoos, 1985).

In 1978 the New York state legislature, encouraged by the success of these early clinics, approved the first state grant to support the development of SBHCs (Making the Grade, 1998). In addition, the newly founded Robert Wood Johnson Foundation, a pioneering supporter for delivering health care for youth through schools, entered the field by funding several school health programs for impoverished children in two communities near Chicago (Isaacs and Knickman, 1999). By the end of the 1970s, fewer than fifty SBHCs had been established across the country, but these early clinics spawned a new approach to health care for youth.

Several developments in the 1980s inspired growth in school-based health centers. Increasing poverty among children, particularly minority youth, led to greater concern about the substantial and myriad problems faced by disadvantaged minors. At the same time the worsening health status among adolescents, especially conditions related to increased sexuality and drug abuse, alarmed both educators and health professionals. High risk for the new morbidities, particularly early childbearing among teens, was the primary rationale for establishing more SBHCs.

The vulnerability of youth to acquiring HIV/AIDS further served to stimulate the development of SBHCs. As summarized by pediatrician and director of the Adolescent AIDS Program at the Montefiore Medical Center, New York City, Karen Hein:

> More than 50 percent of the adolescent girls reported having more than two sexual partners. In various studies, only 25 percent of sexually-active adolescents reported using condoms . . .

As the [AIDS] epidemic spreads *schools, particularly those with health clinics, will have to take greater responsibility for HIV prevention.* (Making the Grade, 1991:1-3) (italics ours)

In 1984, the first national conference of school-based health clinics was held in Houston (TX). It was sponsored by the Center for Population Options (today known as Advocates for Youth) and was attended by representatives from thirty-four SBHCs across the country. Two years later, the Robert Wood Johnson Foundation decided to fund the School-Based Adolescent Health Care Program. This was the first major grant effort focused on replicating comprehensive SBHCs nationwide (Making the Grade, 1998; Dryfoos, 1994).

As innovations in health care, the early school clinics were organized independently yet had common programmatic themes and purposes. Each responded to the growing needs of underserved youth for accessible and confidential health care. Program initiators all believed that schools were the best place to deliver services. Although most SBHCs offered comprehensive health care that ranged from physical examinations to nutrition education, there was a clear emphasis on reproductive services for adolescents. Gynecologic examinations, family planning and sexuality counseling, screening for STDs, and contraceptive prescriptions or referrals to acquire birth control off site were common. Most health services were free, and parental permission to use school clinics was the norm. Furthermore, administrative agencies for SBHCs were quite varied and included hospitals, public health departments, youth agencies, school systems, university medical school programs, and community development agencies. Despite the diversity of organizers, the original model of SBHCs has persisted to the present (Dryfoos, 1994).

EFFECTIVENESS OF SCHOOL-BASED HEALTH CENTERS

In contrast to many other types of school-based prevention programs, school-based health centers have demonstrated effectiveness according to a number of empirical studies. Overall, SBHCs provide access to care for medically underserved youth and increase students' health knowledge significantly. Comprehensive school-based health programs, including SBHCs, have proven successful in increasing utilization of health care, familiarizing students with the health care system, and identifying and treating health problems. High levels of satisfaction have been reported by all groups who are involved with SBHCs, including students, parents, teachers, and school personnel. Characteristics of these centers that are particularly appreciated include their convenience, accessibility, and nurturing staff (Dryfoos, 1994).

Because high-risk health behaviors have been shown to require changes in environment and perceived norms in addition to health knowledge, experts caution that school-based clinics should not—on their own—be expected to change health status or behavior. Nevertheless, SBHCs have reported success in improving contraceptive use, decreasing pregnancy and substance abuse rates, preventing school dropout, and improving school attendance (Allensworth et al., 1997). One study found that students who used SBHCs were twice as likely to stay in school (not drop out) and nearly twice as likely to graduate or be promoted than nonclinic users. In addition, the greater the students' exposure to clinics (actual clinic visits), the higher the graduation or promotion rates. Black males who used SBHCs were three times as likely to stay in school as black male nonusers, and 66 percent of black males who graduated or were promoted were clinic users. Students who visited school health centers were not only staying in school but also succeeding to a greater extent academically, successfully moving ahead to higher grade levels, and fulfilling requirements for graduation (McCord et al., 1993). Another study demonstrated growth in self-esteem and coping skills, improved health and nutritional status, and increased communication with families among students who used the SBHC (Velsor-Friedrich, 1995).

Increasing the access of teens to reproductive health services, and thus the reduction of health problems associated with teen pregnancy and sexually transmitted diseases, have continued to be documented results of SBHC programs. According to Douglas Kirby, a respected authority on both SBHCs and sexuality education issues,

> Since the first school-based health clinic opened in a Dallas high school in 1970, such clinics have been seen not only as a means of providing basic health care to medically underserved teenagers, but as a promising way of addressing some of the intractable and complex health and social problems, particularly

unintended pregnancy, that face young people. (Kirby, Waszak, and Ziegler, 1991:6)

In a more recent analysis (1998), school health care scholar Joy Dryfoos concluded that SBHCs—those that offer comprehensive family-planning services and condom distribution—delay the initiation of sexual intercourse, upgrade the quality of contraceptive use, and lower pregnancy rates. In addition, high proportions of students are being diagnosed and treated for sexually transmitted diseases. Furthermore, comprehensive clinics that reach pregnant and parenting teens demonstrate earlier access to prenatal care and higher birth weights, lower repeat pregnancy rates, and improved school attendance. Most important, in regards to birth control, more than one study has documented that SBHCs that have condoms available improve condom use rates among teens, yet at the same time they do not produce an increase in sexual activity among students in those schools (Schuster et al., 1998).

SBHCs CONFRONT OPPOSITION

Despite their proven effectiveness, the growth of SBHCs sparked the mobilization of conservatives, especially religious fundamentalists, who believed these health care innovations were usurping parental authority by deciding what health and social care was best for children. More significant, conservatives charged that clinics encouraged teenage sexual behavior and abortion and consequently referred to them as "sex clinics." It was this morality issue that most aroused traditional religious groups. In 1986, for example, the Catholic Archbishop of the Los Angeles Diocese strongly criticized the establishment of SBHCs at three high schools in the Los Angeles area. The Archbishop was particularly concerned about the ethical issues posed by the availability of contraceptives to teenagers and by abortion referrals for pregnant girls. In a letter he warned that "by making contraceptives readily available, the clinics' personnel will tacitly promote sexual relations outside of marriage," and he further claimed that abortion was an unacceptable solution to pregnancy (Isaacs and Knickman, 1999:4).

The voices of religious conservatives were strident in a number of locales, and SBHCs were not yet numerous enough to attract national attention. Public officials, especially elected school board members, were sensitive to outcries concerning reproductive care services. As a result, the most controversial of these services—birth control and abortion information and referral—were limited or not provided at all. A 1989 national survey of SBHCs, for example, reported that although 94 percent offered family planning counseling, only 21 percent were actually dispensing some form of birth control on site (Hyche-Williams and Waszak, 1990). No SBHC to date has reported providing, or even wanting to provide, abortion services.

GROWTH OF SBHCS

Beginning with the mid-1980s, school health clinics expanded at a rapid pace. By 1989 there were approximately 150 clinics; two years later this number had more than doubled to 327. Organized primarily in middle and high school and in urban neighborhoods with high rates of poverty, SBHCs had extended into thirty-three states by 1991. Other community youth health centers, many of them school-linked but not actually located within schools, were also proliferating during this time. Yet none of these other approaches to comprehensive health care was as popular or as effective in meeting the needs of children and adolescents. By 1996 school-based clinics numbered 947, almost tripling in the five-year time period from 1991 (Fothergill, 1998). Earlier programs focused mainly on primary care and pregnancy prevention; clinics established in the 1990s addressed a broader range of issues including substance abuse, mental health, and health promotion.

A variety of forces contributed to the dramatic increase in school-based clinics in the late 1980s and 1990s. Growing public awareness of the high levels of poverty and deteriorating health status of American youth was an important factor. This recognition led to greater demand for new approaches to deal with high-risk children and adolescents. The schools were seen as the logical place for health service delivery because, as stated previously, that is where youth are found. In addition, SBHCs were increasingly recognized for their potential to contribute to the national health care reform movement, spurred by economic considerations (health care costs that virtually doubled as a percentage of the national income from 1970 to 1992) as well as by concerns about lack of access to health care (approximately 70 million Americans lacked sufficient health care coverage) (Rosenau, 1994). Many of the medically un- and underinsured were children and adolescents. The health problems suffered by youth in relation to sexual risk behaviors also continued to build support for school-based health centers. In a 1997 report, the Institute of Medicine recommended that "all school districts in the US should ensure that schools provide essential, age-appropriate STD-related services, including health education, access to condoms and *readily accessible and available clinical services, such as school-based clinical services,* to prevent STDs" (quoted in Crosby and St. Lawrence, 2000: 22) (italics ours).

Several significant federal agencies affirmed the potential of SBHCs to address these issues. For example, SBHCs were cited specifically in Healthy People 2000 by the U.S. Public Health Service (1991) as "appropriate" vehicles for reaching youth. A health policy report by the Office of Technology Assessment (1991) heralded SBHCs as "the most promising recent innovation to address the health . . . needs of adolescents" (Making the Grade, 1998:3). In 1994 the General Accounting Office, a nonpartisan research arm of the U.S. Congress, concluded: "SBHCs do improve children's access to health care . . . [through overcoming significant barriers of] lack of health insurance, transportation difficulties, and insufficient attention to the particular needs of adolescents" (1994:1). In addition, health centers in schools had proved capable of overcoming other problems that discouraged youth from utilizing health services, such as inconvenient medical appointments, issues of confidentiality, and prohibitive costs.

There has also been a greater willingness by local and state governments, public health departments and hospitals, universities, and foundations to financially support SBHCs. A number of states have committed to funding SBHCs as part of their efforts in health care reform. By the mid-1990s, for example, more than half the states were providing funds to help organize and extend school-based health centers (Dryfoos, 1994; Fothergill, 1998). Primarily, states have facilitated the ability of clinics to secure reimbursements from Medicaid and managed care organizations. More recently, funds received by states from the federal State Child Health Insurance Program (SCHIP), a program that seeks to expand health insurance coverage to uninsured children, have been utilized by SBHCs (Making the Grade, 1998).

Public support for this new model of health care has been important as well. A 1992 Gallup poll reported that 77 percent of adults surveyed favored the use of public schools as a way to provide health and social services to students. A North Carolina survey a year later showed similar results, with strongest support coming from African Americans and younger adults, presumably those most familiar with SBHCs. Surprisingly, both surveys found that a majority of respondents (60 percent or more) approved of providing birth control at the clinics (Dryfoos, 1994). Another survey, of parents and students in a South Carolina school district, also demonstrated support for the full range of services potentially offered by SBHCs, including reproductive health care (Weathersby, Lobo, and Williamson, 1995). These findings serve as significant testimony to the popularity and degree of support for school health centers and their most controversial services.

SCHOOL CLINICS AS POLICY CHANGE

Most public policy changes at the local level occur in an incremental manner. More radical changes are rare because of the difficulty involved in gaining a consensus among varying interests. Moreover, local policymakers do not often even consider nonincremental changes because such policies are thought to be impossible to implement due to institutional checks and balances. This phenomenon is better known as institutional "gridlock" (Sharp, 1999). In addition to these constraints, some kinds of local policies are more difficult to enact than are others. Perhaps the most difficult are *redistributive* policies that are targeted for the disadvantaged. Essentially, such policies involve taking from those who have resources, usually middle- and upper-class taxpayers, to give to those who have little or none. Such policies are guaranteed to generate resistance and often conflict, especially at the local level where resources are unusually limited (Peterson, 1981).

Given these policy considerations, it is expected that policies designed to implement and fund SBHCs would venture along a treacherous political path. School health clinics are considered nonincremental policies not so much because of the funding allocation (which is typically a relatively modest amount) but because school-based health centers provide health care primarily to poor and minority students. In addition, there is the radical nature of providing reproductive services to youth. The controversy often generated by sexuality—and sometimes other services—means more conflict and debate among larger numbers of interest groups and individuals. Thus gaining the consensus necessary to adopt such a policy becomes ever more difficult. The policy to fund school-based health centers alarms many white middle-class citizens who, for fiscal as well as racial reasons, resent their tax dollars providing care for the "unworthy" children of the community's poor and/or black populace (Stone, 1998). These economic and racial considerations add fuel to the resistance to SBHCs already apparent over the provision of reproductive health care services. Yet despite these significant obstacles to policy adoption and funding, school clinics have grown in number nationwide, even prospering in some states.

POLITICS MATTERS

For a long time a myth has prevailed that "politics and education do not mix" (Wirt and Kirst, 1989:6). Politics often has been viewed as a corrupt process that could only distort and harm the educational system. Thus schools had their own independent governance structure, essentially school boards and superintendents, and financing arrangements. These beliefs and structural organizations served to insulate schools from "outside" politicians and politics more generally.

Although these views of the educational process have always been somewhat naive, the policymaking process in schools has clearly become more politicized in the past several decades. Controversy over policies involving school desegregation, prayer in schools, sexuality education, book censorship, vouchers, inequities in school funding, and accountability have served to expand greatly the role of politics in education. Similarly, the fact that public education has so clearly failed to accomplish its goals for minorities and disadvantaged youth, especially in major cities, has increased interventions into the educational process. Finally, the sheer size of the public investment in elementary and secondary education—about 10 percent of all public spending—increases outsiders' voices and demands in the area of school policy (Stone, 1998).

Thus far there has been little study of health care and politics at the local level. Yet most health services are actually delivered at this level and many new approaches to health care have been developed at the community level. School clinics are one of the more recent innovations. However, most of the research on school-based health centers has focused on their ability to deliver health care services to needy children and adolescents. Numerous studies have explored the planning and implementation of this reform, and the effects of health services on everything from student performance in school to rates of teen pregnancy. Sadly neglected have been the larger and often more important issues that may ultimately determine the future of SBHCs as an educational and health care reform. Inadequate funding and controversy over reproductive services are the visible symptoms of deeper political issues. In the words of political scientist Clarence Stone who has studied school reform, "The question of how to bridge the gap between schools and disadvantaged communities as part of a process of social change brings us face to face with even larger questions about power and social cooperation" (Stone et al., 1998:3). Stone claims that schools, as well as other institutions, cannot carry out reform alone. Meaningful social change requires significant cooperation and assistance from other organizations, groups, and members of the community. None of this collaboration is possible without understanding the politics of social reform, which in this case requires identifying the factors and means needed to harness broad cooperation in the service of disadvantaged and other youth.

OUR STUDY OF SBHCs: WHY IS IT IMPORTANT?

The purpose of this study is to explain how and why this dramatic policy change has occurred, detailing in the process the conditions and strategies that have proven helpful in the success of SBHCs. This book presents the results of our investigation of the factors that affect the establishment and maintenance of this important innovation in education and health care delivery. While we explore SBHC provision of health and social services generally, we are especially interested in reproductive health care, the most controversial yet perhaps the most needed services. Among the factors of possible importance to clinic maintenance, we focus on the nature and degree of school and community support, political opposition, role of the media, state-level support, available funding sources, student health needs, and the political climate. Clearly our emphasis is on the politics of school-based health centers, a long-neglected area of concern and of utmost importance to the creation, longevity, and success of SBHCs.

Our study of SBHCs utilizes a two-pronged approach: a nation-wide survey of clinic administrators supplemented with aggregate data, and intensive case studies of five representative locales. The combination of quantitative data from a national survey and more qualitative information gathered from case study fieldwork permits us to offer broad generalizations as well as to report the meaning of our findings in more detail.

In 1998 we surveyed a random sample (N = 350) of all SBHCs (N = 1,153) based on the national census conducted by the National Assembly on School-Based Health Care. The survey focused on the politics of community involvement and support for school-based clinics. With a response rate of 74 percent (after adjusting the sample for nonclinics and closed clinics), we produced information on a valid representative sample of all SBHCs. Analysis of these data supplemented with aggregate information on each community allowed us to develop models of the life history of clinics, especially the effects of hostile and supportive environments. The responses of clinic directors to open-ended questions were especially useful in defining the important problems, as well as successful strategies, of SBHCs across the country.

Our other important source of information comes from in-depth case studies of five representative, diverse (geographically, ethnically, and by sources of funding) sites across the United States. These sites were selected on the basis of our 1991 national survey of school-based clinics and were studied in depth as part of our first look at the politics of SBHC development conducted in the early 1990s (Rienzo and Button, 1993; Rienzo, 1994). In 1998-1999 we returned to these settings to see how the SBHCs have evolved. The information gleaned from these case studies provides an important longitudinal dimension for this study. These representative sites are located in the following cities and settings:

- Albuquerque, NM (East San Jose Elementary School, a poor Latino urban neighborhood setting);
- Jersey City, NJ (Snyder High School, a poor African-American and Latino inner-city school);
- Portland, OR (Parkrose High School, a white middle-class suburban school);
- Quincy, FL (Shanks High School, a poor, largely African-American school located in the rural South);
- Virginia Beach, VA (a white, middle-class urban area where the effort to establish an SBHC has been thwarted successfully by opponents).

In both the early and late 1990s, we interviewed in each community a variety of respondents considered knowledgeable about clinic evolution and politics. These individuals typically included clinic directors and staff, school administrators, teachers, parents, school board members, clinic advisory board members, leaders of community groups both supportive and in opposition to clinics, and media representatives. Local newspapers and available clinic records added further insight into these case studies.

In terms of the format of this book, in Chapter 2 we look at the most serious problems and barriers confronted by school health centers, and why some SBHCs have closed. In particular the issues of funding, lack of parental and community support, religious-based opposition, conflicts between health professionals and educators, and other problems mentioned by clinic directors are analyzed. Political conflicts involving race and poverty and the redistribution of health services are important general issues that are examined. We illustrate these problems with reference to our case studies in Virginia Beach, Jersey City, and Quincy, as well as drawing upon information from our survey. This analysis explains why some SBHCs are unsuccessful (deliver few services, are poorly funded, have little community support) and why others close or never get started despite the demand for youth health services.

Chapter 3 explores in detail the factors that have enabled some SBHCs to grow, develop, and flourish. We look at how health clinics in schools get started, and how they maintain themselves, dealing successfully with funding, controversy, and other issues. Focusing on our case studies, we chronicle the success achieved by SBHCs in

Portland and Albuquerque. Our national survey of clinics enables us to develop generalizations about the political and other factors that contribute to the growth and development of SBHCs.

Chapter 4 discusses the politics of reproductive services, the most controversial element of school health centers. Teenagers in the United States have the highest pregnancy rates and birthrates of any such age group in the Western industrialized world. Thus a tremendous need exists for reproductive and family planning services, and most SBHCs at the middle and high school levels attempt to address these issues. However, the salience of sexual behavior and services is a highly charged "morality politics" issue that often overwhelms attempts to frame it as a public health concern. This chapter focuses on the political opposition to reproductive health care, especially to contraception availability. We explore the nature of the opposition, their political tactics, and why they are often successful in limiting or, in some cases, prohibiting sexuality-related services. Political strategies for successfully countering opponents are described. Again, we draw upon each of our case studies and the national survey to provide analysis and illustrations.

Finally, our book concludes with Chapter 5, in which we summarize our results and make recommendations for developing and sustaining school health centers. We explore major issues that still confront many SBHCs as they continue to grow and develop. These issues include financial support, adding mental health services, dealing with sexual orientation, the "gender gap" in providing services, the neglect of needy Latino students, underutilized resources, accountability, and contending with racial barriers. For each issue, we suggest ways to successfully deal with the problem. Finally, we return to our theme of "politics as the key" to developing these and other school reforms.

Chapter 2

Major Problems
of School Health Centers

Views of "at-risk" youth, as well as approaches to working with them, are extremely varied. These range from wanting to provide additional services to a more punitive approach. These views serve as a barrier to developing comprehensive plans for issues such as sexuality, violence, drugs, and alcohol.

SBHC director, Portsmouth, NH

In 20 percent of the nation's approximately 80,000 schools, more than half of the students are so poor that they qualify for federally subsidized meals. Many health professionals, educators, and others believe that these roughly 16,000 schools dominated by poverty-stricken youth should be of high priority in the movement toward school-based clinics and other forms of full service schools (Dryfoos, 1994). Yet despite the dramatic increase in SBHCs in the 1990s, only about 1,400 clinics are presently in operation.

Although school health centers have received broad support from almost every national health and social service organization, the collaborative arrangements necessary to establish and maintain SBHCs are not easily achieved. In our national survey, clinic coordinators listed numerous factors that play a role in inhibiting the maintenance and growth of their health centers. The most frequently listed were lack of funding, including problems with third-party reimbursement and managed care organizations; political opposition from conservative groups; staff shortages and lack of trained personnel; general ignorance of and false beliefs about clinic services; lack of state support; competition from other health and human service providers; lack of parental awareness and support, as well as parents' concerns about reproductive services; and insufficient support from school boards and school personnel.

In this chapter, we discuss these important barriers to the establishment and growth of SBHCs. We also explore the underlying conditions or more fundamental problems that plague school clinics. Finally, we will take a close look at three school districts where school health centers either proved to be less than successful over time (Quincy, FL, and Jersey City, NJ) or failed altogether in the preliminary stage of development (Virginia Beach, VA). In each case, various political factors were important in the demise of the clinics.

DAY-TO-DAY ISSUES

Numerous problems affect many school clinics on a daily basis. Shortages of staff and space, lack of support from teachers and parents, budget shortfalls, and controversy over reproductive services are typical challenges that confront clinic personnel regularly. Our research has indicated that some of these day-to-day issues are a greater hindrance to the success of SBHCs than other factors. It is important to discern which of these issues are most significant and how they afflict school clinics.

Inadequate and Unstable Funding

The most important issue identified by directors of school health centers is long-term funding. Annual costs of a clinic range between $100,000 and $300,000, depending on the size of the school and the range of services offered. Foundations or state initiatives typically provide start-up costs in the form of demonstration grants that cover the first three to five years. After this initial period, however, long-term and consistent sources of support are difficult to acquire. Indeed, in our national survey of clinic coordinators, lack of funding was by far the most frequently mentioned barrier (62 percent) to SBHC maintenance and growth. As a clinic director in Oakland (CA) stated, "Funding is *always* a problem. The kids who come to the clinic almost by definition cannot pay for the services and do not have insurance. We run approximately $10,000 in the red each year, which is offset by foundation grants and some county dollars, but it's a struggle."

Beyond the first years of development, SBHCs must often rely on a variety of funding sources to maintain or add services. School health centers therefore have to deal with multiple financing arrangements, learn to capture reimbursements from third-party insurance and Medicaid, and overcome the hurdles of managed care. The rapid growth of managed care in the 1990s, driven by the effort to contain health care costs, has posed particularly difficult challenges for many SBHCs. Based on capitated funding, managed care plans often do not cover the full array of comprehensive services offered by school-based clinics. Nonmedical yet important preventive services such as health or sexuality education, mental health services, and health screening tend not to be included. Managed care contracts typically limit the choice of provider, often omitting SBHCs which reduces students' access to critically needed services. Many SBHCs have been delayed in, or blocked from, integrating into managed care systems, and states are just beginning to support (through mandate or enhanced compensation) the inclusion of school-based clinics in this restructuring of the health care system (Dryfoos, 1994; Santelli et al., 1998). For example, in 1998, only 28 percent of school health centers had worked out formal relationships with managed care organizations, and only 50 percent of these clinics reported being full primary care providers (Fothergill, 1998).

One of the most common sources of funding for SBHCs is third-party reimbursement, usually Medicaid, since most clinic users come from poor families. Despite being a popular source, only 12 percent of health center budgets are obtained from this billing. This low level of funding has largely been due to the fact that only 28 percent of SBHC users have Medicaid coverage even though many more are eligible. Lack of awareness of Medicaid and how to obtain coverage are the primary barriers, with the lowest rates of participation found in rural areas and among black and Hispanic youth (Fothergill, 1998).

In addition, Medicaid recipients are increasingly required to join managed care organizations, which have their own set of problems regarding SBHCs. To help rectify this situation, the federal government enacted the State Children's Health Insurance Program (SCHIP) in 1997, allocating $4 billion annually for ten years to states to expand health insurance coverage for children up to age eighteen. The largest initiative of its kind, states are able to use the funds to enlarge Medicaid programs or to create other health insurance plans for children. Nonetheless, after three years of this program effort, states had not enrolled many new families, with 60 percent of parents whose children lack health insurance claiming they did not know about the program ("Many Eligible Families Lack Health Benefits," 2000). In Florida, for example, there are an estimated 372,000 uninsured youth that are eligible for SCHIP, but only 144,000 had been enrolled by mid-2000. The state, similar to many others, may lose a substantial portion of its SCHIP funding because of its inability to provide health insurance to poor children ("Poor Kids May Never See Funds," 2000).

Lack of Visible Parental Support and Involvement

Although parental support for school-based provision of health services and education is vitally important, such support is not always certain, especially when controversy develops over clinical services such as reproductive health care for adolescents. In fact, parents' voices "are rarely heard above the noisy rhetoric of conservative pressure groups" that claim to be speaking on their behalf (Dryfoos and Santelli, 1992:259). Although local surveys of youth health needs could provide much needed parental support for clinics, such assessments are rarely conducted. As a result, the full complement of services clinics might provide to meet the needs of students has often been constrained (Weathersby, Lobo, and Williamson, 1995).

Ideally, parents are engaged at multiple levels in the SBHC structure in addition to their children's participation: as clinic aides, paid workers, advisory board members, and sometimes as patients (Allensworth et al., 1997). However, school-based clinics have experienced a range of barriers when attempting to involve parents. Some parents feel threatened due to a fear of being blamed for their child's problems, while others see SBHC staff as unwanted interference in maintaining control over their child's health. Problems involving families also are logistical in nature, such as matching the schedules of working parents with clinic hours, lack of transportation, and unavailability of child care in the home (Bickham et al., 1998; Dryfoos, 1994). In other cases parents are simply unaware of a school health center because poverty-ridden adults often lack basic information about their communities.

More recent issues relate to those parents who are not U.S. citizens and who therefore lack access to state or federal medical reimbursement, feel threatened to legal exposure, and/or have cultural beliefs that conflict with Western medical care. These problems were affirmed by clinic coordinators in their responses to a question regarding barriers to growth and success on our national survey. Their comments about these issues included: "Hispanic cultural beliefs in alternative medicines and low use of traditional health care" (AZ); "Not allowing those families who have no health insurance to access our services" (HI); and "The fear of parents to reveal any information about themselves or their kids due to their undocumented status" (NY).

Unsupportive Teachers, School Administrators, or School Boards

A crucial component to SBHC development is the active support of the inner circle comprised of school officials and teachers. Not gaining this support will significantly deter or completely obstruct the institutionalization of clinic operations. Leadership by school officials and school board members is crucial to clinic success. Without the leadership of key power holders, there is no catalyst to bring people together to collaborate around the needs of disadvantaged children. Many school officials are not willing to take the political risks necessary to support health services that are often controversial and require additional monies. In addition, many school systems are so overburdened with demands for academic improvement that they ignore initiatives that seemingly have nothing to do with enhancing the educational program (Doherty, Jones, and Stone, 1998). According to a survey response by a Wisconsin SBHC coordinator, the foremost barrier to his clinic was "a school board and school administration (at the central office level) that neither understands nor appreciates the health needs of students."

Support within the school is just as critical as leadership in the community. The principal establishes policy, which the teachers enact, that enables (or hinders) students to access the school clinic. Results of a recent survey found that "many teachers are unfamiliar with school-based health centers and the services they provide. . . . It's important that the teachers know about the availability of services because the teachers are critical referral points" (Making the Grade, 1999:2). Often teachers perceive that they must compete with SBHCs for space, if it is in short supply, and for students' time when they miss classroom instruction to visit the clinic. Moreover, school personnel most sensitive to the lack of health care for poor students and supportive of school health centers are minority members and those who live in or near poverty-ridden neighborhoods. Most school personnel, however, are white, live in middle-class residential areas, and are often insensitive to the needs of minority students (Emihovich and Herrington, 1997).

Staff Shortages and Training

The growth of school-based health centers has been limited by an acute shortage of personnel. Indeed, based on our national survey, SBHC directors listed this fifth most frequently as a factor inhibiting the expansion of school clinics. The only issues mentioned more often were problem areas involving funding and political opposition to SBHCS. The typical clinic employs a full-time nurse practitioner, social worker, receptionist, and community aide and often has the part-time services of a pediatrician, psychologist, health educator, nutritionist, or substance abuse counselor. The nurse practitioner (NP) is the primary coordinator in most SBHCs, and NPs are in great demand in a variety of community health programs and private physicians' practices (Dryfoos, 1994). Mental health services are the fastest-growing component of school health centers, according to our survey, and social workers and other professionals who provide such services are also in short supply.

The lack of health care professionals is only part of the problem. At least as important an issue is the particular cross-discipline training necessary for clinic directors. Such persons must be able to bridge the professional fields of health, psychology, social development, and education. Furthermore, clinic coordinators need to know how to obtain and manage multiple sources of funds; work well with students, parents, teachers, and school administrators; manage a wide range of professional staff; be accountable to community agencies; and help build community, school, and local political support for their health centers. Other key clinic personnel must be able to play many of these roles as well.

Training health center staff to deal effectively with children and adolescents in times of crisis and to deal with conditions related to dire poverty is a challenge as well. As an Albuquerque (NM) school official and advocate of SBHCs put it, "It's difficult to find properly trained personnel to deal with ever-changing issues, like mental health problems resulting from low socioeconomic status. Our community has real poverty, crime, drugs, and alcohol abuse that most people never see, and universities don't train professionals for this" (Interview, May 5, 1999). As an example of the unusual medical situations confronting SBHC staff, a nurse at an elementary school clinic in New Mexico told us of a poor Latino boy who complained of chronic pain in an ear. When the health center physician examined the youth, he was shocked to find a dead roach in the child's ear. The boy revealed that his family was so large and poor that he slept on the floor where roaches run freely (Interview, May 1, 1992). As a result of health issues for which they are not always prepared, as well as having heavy caseloads of underserved youth, clinics experience a high staff turnover rate.

Turf Wars

A school health center director in Milwaukee (WI) claimed that one of the major conflicts affecting her clinic was "a local group of physicians and managed care organizations that see SBHCs as competition and not as complements to their services" (response to our national survey). Any time a new health care reform or agency is introduced, there will be inevitable conflict with some existing health service providers. For example, medical doctors, especially pediatricians, sometimes object that school clinics take away potential patients. School nurses also typically feel displaced by SBHCs, as do many school counselors, social workers, and psychologists when a full-service clinic is operative. Moreover, these other professionals often want access to student information obtained through the clinic. However, due to the confidential nature of such information, working relationships among the various professionals require careful planning regarding how and whether such information is disseminated (Dryfoos, 1998; Hacker and Wessel, 1998).

Turf wars appear as well when outside agency-governed health providers are brought into a school system which has policies and practices that become barriers to community-based professionals. Health and school staffs operate under separate authorities, each with their own unions, pay schedules, hours of work, and direction. A major area of potential conflict is the school's rules of discipline. The school has its own policies, such as suspension and other forms of punishment, that may run counter to the beliefs of "newcomers" who are more focused on the emotional and physical needs of students. Teachers in particular may oppose SBHCs when students leave classes for clinic appointments. In addition, there is often competition for space, especially in schools that are run-down and over-crowded. Health centers require several rooms that are safe and secure to provide even basic services in a confidential manner. Center staff also make demands on school resources for maintenance, security, cleaning services, and additional hours in which the school is open for access to the clinic. These demands can be expensive, and the schools that typically house clinics are the ones least able to afford such additional costs (Allensworth et al., 1997; Dryfoos, 1998; Hacker and Wessel, 1998; Flaherty et al., 1998).

Cultural Issues

The majority of students (and their parents) served by SBHCs are poor and minority, primarily African American and Hispanic, while most clinic staff are middle-class and white. This situation typically produces a substantial cultural divide. In one Florida SBHC it was reported that minority parents viewed information about diet as "a culturally-biased attack on (their) family eating habits" (Emihovich and Herrington, 1997:163). Our investigation of the East San Jose Elementary School health center revealed that some cultural tension existed between white middle-class doctors and nurses and lower-class Hispanic students. In the words of one Latino school official, "some whites in the clinic appear arrogant and are not trusted" by students (Interview, May 5, 1999). As a result of this perception, students were less likely to visit the health center.

Cultural differences can create serious conflicts as well as an atmosphere of distrust and misunderstanding. Many health care providers in SBHCs are neither culturally sensitive nor aware, often not speaking the language of minority students nor having a working knowledge of their culture. Few professional schools require foreign language study or cultural diversity training as part of the medical or health education curriculum (Interview, New Mexico state official, May 5, 1999). Yet public schools are increasingly populated by nonwhite and sometimes non–English-speaking minorities as immigration to the United States and minority birthrates remain at high levels. This is particularly an issue for elementary SBHCs, where consultation with parents is essential for the care of their children.

Cultural gaps are especially noticeable in SBHC attempts to deal with issues related to teenage sexuality. To avoid possible conflict and controversy, health center personnel generally avoid frank and open discussions of sexuality. This is in stark contrast to most adolescents who are repeatedly exposed to explicit messages about sexual activity from peers, the media, and the Internet. When clinic staff do talk about sexual issues, they are often framed in a white, middle-class perspective. For example, teenage pregnancy is typically cast as a serious barrier to success in later life. Yet for poor black and Latino girls with few career or other life-enhancing prospects, having a child is often an affirmation of their adult status. In other controversial areas of sexuality, such as issues regarding adolescent abortion and homosexuality, school health personnel are often totally silent. Not only do they face enormous societal constraints in discussing these issues, but many clinic staff are severely limited by their middle-class bias that such behaviors are morally wrong, abnormal, and/or deviant (Emihovich and Herrington, 1997).

Lack of Assessment and Evaluation Data

A problem for many SBHC advocates is the dearth of evidence that school health centers really "work." Myriad problems have been identified that influence this issue, including the mobility of low-income populations, inadequate methods to measure outcomes (i.e., pregnancy rates), and the high cost of effective evaluation procedures to account for long-term and preventive results. The Institute of Medicine (Allensworth et al., 1997) assessment of the limited solid research that exists on effectiveness of school clinics concluded that health centers could be successfully implemented in schools, enroll substantial numbers of students, provide adequate care in a cost-effective manner, and were perceived positively by users with respect to quality of services and providers. Nonetheless, the paucity of "hard data" proving SBHCs' influence on specific desirable outcomes, such as decreased pregnancy and birthrates among teenagers, is a significant barrier to their growth and acceptance (Dryfoos, 1994; Allensworth et al., 1997).

The lack of good outcome evidence enables the opposition to make claims about the negative (or lack of) effects of SBHCs without being adequately challenged. As noted by a survey respondent from Arkansas, "The false information that's given out regarding school clinics [is a barrier], and the true benefits or positive benefits are very seldom known or shared by the media." Moreover, without sound evaluation data parents and educators may hesitate to support or recommend SBHCs, and students may be more reluctant to use them.

MAJOR UNDERLYING ISSUES

Although there has been much discussion of the more obvious day-to-day issues confronting many school-based clinics, there has been almost total disregard, misunderstanding, and naïveté concerning the major underlying problems. Countless studies and articles have focused on issues such as inadequate staff, need for Medicaid or third-party reimbursements, competition with other health care providers, and lack of visible community or parental support. To be sure, all these are factors that affect the growth and development of SBHCs. Yet each of these issues is often the result of deeper conflicts and concerns that are at the root of problems plaguing school clinics and other school reforms. Until these more fundamental problems are understood and addressed, the persistent symptoms that become a chronic nuisance will never be fully alleviated.

School Reformers versus Health Providers

One of the deep-seated dilemmas confronting SBHCs is how to integrate this new form of child and adolescent health care with school reform movements that are changing educational systems. School reforms are varied, but the recent focus has been on raising student academic achievement by setting national educational standards. Most of the debate about school reform involves two different approaches: school reorganization which is a model of change of the whole school system, and targeted school interventions which would identify high-risk students and offer programs to change their lives and enhance educational achievement. This latter reform effort is more in the mode of SBHCs with "add-on" programs focusing on issues such as dropout prevention, substance abuse prevention, or educational enhancement. Other models of school reform do not provide for health and human services in the schools (Dryfoos, 1998).

Most school reformers are concerned with school reorganization, curriculum design, test scores, and teacher training. Health care is sometimes perceived as a needless dilution of the school's intellectual mission. This view is increasingly seen as naive, however, as reformers are more often linking student success with ready access to health and social services (Dryfoos, 1994; Making the Grade, 1993). Yet it is unclear as to how to best provide these necessary health services, and how they might be included in a full service school without detracting from academic emphases. There is also fear that financing comprehensive health services will take away funding from more important educational programs. As a result, school reformers and health care advocates are often at odds. Until this conflict is resolved, school health centers will be perceived as costly, fringe, or unnecessary services that do not belong in the schools of the future.

Fiscal Constraints of American Cities

Most school health centers (61 percent) are found in urban areas. While SBHCs provide nontraditional health care to large numbers of medically uninsured youths, thus creating significant financial woes for most clinics, local governments exist under their own set of serious fiscal constraints. Dillon's Rule, a nineteenth-century legal decision that limits the tax powers of cities, has restricted local revenues including those of school districts. More recently, tax revolts and public initiatives have forced local officials to keep taxes low. Most important, the shift of industry and middle-class residents from cities to suburbs over the past fifty years has eroded the inner-city tax base. Those who remain in the central city tend to be poorer and require more services, thus driving up expenditures. Even higher tax rates yield low revenues in cities depleted of their wealth.

Inner-city schools have become particularly disadvantaged. As educational requirements for good jobs are rising, the quality of education available in the center city has been eroded by the concentration of children from poverty-ridden families. At the same time the financial and educational disparity between inner-city and more affluent suburban schools has become greater. With the maintenance of separate school districts for central cities and suburbs, a serious mismatch between needs and resources has resulted. Coupled with little federal assistance for schools in general, and with many states that are reluctant to grant greater funds for deteriorating inner-city schools, the fiscal picture for urban education is bleak (Dye, 2000; Kweit and Kweit, 1999).

Added to these fiscal limitations are the new and costly responsibilities placed on schools. Class sizes have grown intolerably large; there is a great need for school construction, expansion, and renovation; computer and related technology demands are enormous; and restructuring efforts have required increased resources (Emihovich and Herrington, 1997). As a result, school health centers receive limited amounts of support from city governments or school districts and must compete with dozens of other worthwhile projects for scarce community agency funds. Such daunting financial problems prevent many sites from even considering the creation of an SBHC; in other locations, maintaining a fledgling health clinic after the initial foundation or other start-up funding ceases is a major challenge.

Politics of Race and Class

Social scientists Michael Danielson and Jennifer Hochshield (1998) claim:

> Race and class, and their interaction, have more impact on education than on any other major public function. With a few celebrated exceptions, the quality and effectiveness of public schools are strongly related to the class (and therefore usually to the race) of the students in a particular school or district. (281)

Tensions created by race are particularly pronounced in education because of the history of desegregation. The brutal struggles to desegregate schools and create greater equality in education have left a legacy of distrust and anxiety between many blacks (and more recently Hispanics) and whites.

Thus strains due to race and class conflicts have often thwarted collaborative initiatives, including those to create and sustain school health clinics. SBHCs provide health care for children and adolescents who need it most, which means primarily poor African-American and Hispanic youth. However, the economic means necessary to develop school health centers must come primarily from the white community. Although blacks and Hispanics have gained political power, especially in larger American cities, the business community, which is heavily white, maintains economic control. Moreover, the informal relationships between races that are necessary to build mutual trust are noticeably absent. Race and class divide not only cities and suburbs, but cities have also seen their political influence at the state level decline as the power of the suburbs has grown (Doherty et al., 1998; Rich, 1996).

Increasingly an "us versus them" mentality has developed between racial minorities and whites. In the case of school health center reproductive services, a recent survey of South Carolina voters showed that whites and those economically well off are less likely to be supportive than are blacks and the poor (Lindley, Reininger, and Saunders, 2001). For many whites it seems that too many resources are directed to minority populations, and for many black and Hispanics it appears that their neighborhoods are the areas of greatest need and therefore require more resources. Public schools, moreover, hold a special place for racial minorities for it is a policy area that is strongly associated with the promise of greater opportunity and a place where their demands will be heard (Stone, 1998).

Social class divisions exacerbate racial divisions. Income has always been severely maldistributed in the United States. Since 1947 the poorest 20 percent of American families have received less than 5 percent of before-tax income annually, while the richest 20 percent have consistently received over 40 percent of all before-tax income. The distribution of wealth (income plus assets) much more heavily favors the rich (Rodgers, 1979). In terms of race, blacks and Hispanics have always had much higher rates of poverty than whites. In 1990, for example, the poverty rate among blacks was 32 percent; for Hispanics, 28 percent; and among whites, 11 percent (U.S. Bureau of the Census, 1990). In terms of actual numbers, however, most poor people in this country are white, yet many Americans perceive poverty as primarily a problem mainly confronting racial and ethnic minorities.

In addition, there has been and continues to be strong public support for the belief that the individual is primarily responsible for his or her own economic conditions. Institutional or structural causes of poverty, such as lack of jobs and poor conditions of the nation's public schools, are considered less important than individualistic factors such as immoral behavior, substance abuse, and lack of effort by the poor themselves. Consistent with this view, Americans show a relatively weak commitment to most public programs to reduce poverty. When poor blacks are considered, overwhelming majorities of whites are opposed to government economic assistance. Attitudes of white racism merge with an emphasis on individualism to undermine support for social programs for African Americans (Bobo and Smith, 1994). Although these public attitudes are not inflexible and vary somewhat depending on the public policy proposed, they do provide political constraints on policies affecting poor and racial minorities.

Culture War Politics

One of the most visible and significant conflicts faced by advocates of school-based health centers involves morality politics. This domain of public policy is distinctive because the issues engage the fundamental values and moral concerns of citizens. Schools have long been a political battleground of contested values over issues such as prayer, desegregation, sex education, teaching the concept of evolution, and the censorship of books. These issues typically create a great deal of conflict because they raise the kind of values-based concerns about right and wrong that make it difficult for opposing groups to find common ground and compromise. So divisive are many of these political battles over moral issues that they are likened to a culture war (Hunter, 1991).

Clearly the politics of providing reproductive services in school health centers is a morally contentious issue. Among their primary goals, clinics address issues of reproductive health care, particularly high rates of teen pregnancy and sexually transmitted diseases (STDs). In attempting to reduce both epidemics, many SBHCs provide services ranging from sexuality education to access to birth control, including condoms, abortion counseling and referral, and testing and treatment for STDs, including HIV.

The salience of sexual behavior in American political discourse usually overwhelms any attempt to frame such services strictly in terms of public health. In many communities, the opponents of clinics have emphasized SBHCs' alleged endorsement of teen sexual activity by labeling them as "sex" or "abortion" clinics (Dryfoos, 1994). In New York City, Joseph Fernandez, chancellor of schools and one of the foremost educators in the country, was forced to resign in the early 1990s in the wake of a controversy over sexuality in the curriculum and making condoms available to high school students (Emihovich and Herrington, 1997). The most consistent and strident opposition to school clinics has come from conservative Protestants and, to a lesser extent, the Catholic Church. For these religious groups SBHCs represent a pernicious public policy that promotes sexual promiscuity and lack of respect for traditional values. In their efforts to block or close school health centers, these groups have often used the tactics of a culture war, portraying the conflict as a clash of moral absolutes with major consequences for society (Rienzo and Button, 1993).

CHARACTERISTICS OF LESS SUCCESSFUL CLINICS

Why do some school health centers close, others never get started, and a number fail to provide many services or even begin to meet the needs of disadvantaged students? One recent survey of SBHCs in six western states estimated that 10 percent of clinics had ceased to operate after less than two years of providing services (Johnston, 1998). Our own national survey indicates that approximately 5 percent of once-viable school health centers have closed their doors. These attrition rates are relatively large. We have no way of knowing how many other clinics failed to open at all even when youth health needs were apparent and advocates had hoped to initiate an SBHC.

We are able to provide some answers about why some SBHCs are relatively unsuccessful in offering many services, staying open a sufficient number of hours each day, and/or attracting enough students to utilize the clinic. Looking at the results of our national survey and the composite measure of success, or lack of success in this case, we can describe the clinics that are failing as viable, vibrant school health centers (Rienzo, Button, and Wald, 2000). These clinics scored in the lowest tenth percentile on our composite index and thus represent a clear contrast to the characteristics of most centers (Table 2.1).

The most compelling characteristic of the least successful SBHCs is that they are found primarily in rural settings (76 percent) rather

TABLE 2.1. General Characteristics of Least Successful SBHCs

	Least Successful (N = 22)	Average (N = 183)
Community Demographics		
Size of city (in thousands)	373	417
Percent African American	14	20
Percent Hispanic	14	13
Income	$12,115	$13,347
Percent poverty	18	19
Local percent Clinton vote, 1996	53	56
Percent college education	16	19
Percent conservative Protestants	23	23
School Characteristics		
Minority school board officials	<1	4
School enrollment	865	1,134
Percent black enrollment	19	34
Percent Hispanic enrollment	17	19
Percent enrollment on free/reduced lunch	55	61
SBHC Characteristics		
Annual budget (1997-1998)	$38,800	$133,680
Percent users of clinic	45	62
Percent non-Hispanic white users	56	40
Percent within state association of SBHCs	30	41

than in urban or suburban locales. Unlike urban-based school clinics, these rural health centers provide services for largely non-Hispanic white students (an average of 56 percent). Although these mainly white youth are disadvantaged, with 55 percent qualifying for the free or reduced federal lunch program, they are not as needy as the primarily minority youth found in urban schools, where 66 percent are eligible to participate in the government-sponsored lunch program. With blacks constituting only 19 percent of the students in these rural schools, and Hispanics only 17 percent, minority youth with the highest health risk behaviors are relatively small in proportions. Small minority populations translate into relatively few black and Hispanic school board members, who often are among the strongest advocates of SBHCs. All of this in turn creates a smaller demand for clinical services, as 45 percent of students enrolled in the clinics actually used services in the mostly rural schools. This compares with a 73 percent SBHC usage rate in largely minority, urban schools.

Another factor that distinguished these less successful health centers was their statewide political environment. Most of these SBHCs are located in conservative Sunbelt and southern border states, including Arkansas, Arizona, Georgia, New Mexico, Tennessee, and West Virginia. Clinics in these states faced greater opposition, especially from religious groups, and had less support from community organizations than health centers elsewhere. Furthermore, relatively few of these rural clinics (30 percent) belonged to statewide associations of SBHCs, which are potentially helpful in building support at the state level. As articulated by a clinic director in rural Louisiana in response to our national survey question about barriers to SBHC growth and development:

> We are located in a very "right-wing" area where politics are based on Christian values and the Christian Coalition has a huge influence on politicians at the state level. Our state senator is very conservative, influenced a lot by the Christian Coalition, and is totally opposed to health centers.

In addition, there was almost no consistent communication with the media among these unsuccessful health centers, which meant that little or no publicity about the activities of the clinics was being generated. For many of these SBHCs, however, it was a matter of confronting more than simply one or two barriers; often a host of problems plagued these clinics. "We face staff turnover, staff conflicts with each other, poor outcomes (evaluation) measures, unclear program objectives, and not enough community and media outreach," commented a rural North Carolina clinic coordinator in response to our survey.

Lack of success was most clearly apparent in the extremely low level of funding and the absence of consistent, stable financial support. Clinic directors in our survey cited insufficient funding as the chief obstacle confronting most SBHCs. Yet for the least successful health centers, this issue was critical. Average annual funding was a meager $39,000 (almost $100,000 below the national median), which kept clinic doors open only fourteen hours a week during the school year and closed in the summer. Although serious financial problems are an obvious indicator that centers are in trouble, they are in reality a symptom of deeper ills affecting such clinics.

Quincy (FL): Crisis of Black Youth in the Deep South

Located just south of the Georgia border in rural north Florida, Quincy is the quintessential small, southern community. It is nestled in the land of Dixie where King Cotton and tobacco once reigned supreme in a plantation system supported by slave labor. Even today African Americans make up a majority of Gadsden County's population, and the "southern way of life," including Civil War memories and issues of race and poverty, permeate the culture (Button, 1989).

In 1985, Dr. Philip Porter, of Harvard University's School of Public Health and also of the Robert Wood Johnson Foundation (RWJ), was invited by the Gadsden County Health Department to visit Quincy to investigate severe adolescent health problems. Porter, founder of one of the nation's first SBHCs in Cambridge (MA), discovered a community whose youth were in crisis (Fiedler, 1986). A 1985 survey of students at Shanks High School in Quincy (the city's only public high school) indicated that approximately 90 percent of students were black; over 50 percent reported they were sexually active; 90 percent had no access to routine health care; and the teen birthrate was second highest among the state's sixty-seven counties (*Final Report,* 1995). In addition, 80 percent of Shanks' students qualified for free or reduced lunches, suggesting the pressing poverty that had long plagued the community. Often beset by a host of problems, many students either gave up on or dropped out of school (Fiedler, 1986).

At about the same time that Porter appeared, the local council of the Governor's Constituency For Children, a group of community leaders appointed by Governor Bob Graham (D), began to hold public forums on adolescent health. The forums proved informative, and the local council agreed that the single most important health issue was the unusually high rate of teen pregnancies ("Clinic Concept Is Praiseworthy," 1985). As a result of the local council's activities and the growing community concern over youth health problems and teen pregnancy, a formal coalition was formed to plan strategies to improve health services. The community coalition included representatives from health and social service agencies, schools, community-based programs, parent groups, the ministerial association, and concerned citizens (*Final Report,* 1995; Interviews, April 8, 10, 1992).

With advice from Porter, the coalition proposed a school-based health center for Shanks High School. School and health officials were aware that the only source of health care for students was the county health department located several miles from school and outside of the city. Most students had no transportation; for them, the health department was inaccessible. When students did gain permission to leave school to go to the health department, they often did not return to school. Public health officials strongly supported the establishment of an SBHC to make health services more readily available to teenagers (Interviews, April 8, 10, 1992).

In late 1985, a planning committee composed of local health and social service providers developed a grant proposal for a Shanks clinic. The school principal and county superintendent of schools were very supportive. Florida State University and Florida A & M College in nearby Tallahassee offered expertise and planning resources, and RWJ and the national Center for Population Options contributed technical assistance. Also important, community support was broad and included school officials, teachers, parents, ministers, women's groups, physicians, hospital officials, and local government leaders. Formal approval of the school health center by the county commission and school board came relatively quickly and easily (Wooten 1985b; Interviews, April 8, 10, 1992). In December, initial start-up funds of $47,000 for the clinic came from the state's Maternal and Child Health block grant (*Final Report,* 1995).

During public discussions of the proposed SBHC only a few local citizens voiced opposition. Their concern focused on the plan to provide birth control prescriptions and devices on site. "The clinics will encourage immorality," charged one opponent who feared similar clinics would be placed in other schools (Washington, 1986:1). Advocates countered these concerns by emphasizing that parental permission was required for students to receive any clinic services, and that birth control was only one of many health services to be offered (Wooten, 1985a).

Once the health center opened in 1986 at Shanks High School, however, stronger opposition from outside the county began to mobilize. The Catholic Conference, based in Tallahassee, the Big Bend Right to Life Organization of north Florida, and the Freedom Council, the political arm of Pat Robertson's Christian Coalition which was located in Virginia Beach, all moved to block or limit clinic activities. Members of these organizations attended public meetings, wrote letters to the local newspaper, and even picketed outside the school. Proponents of the health center publicly responded that "outsiders" were trying to dictate policy for local schools, and this tactic served to solidify the community against the opposition (*Final Report,* 1995; Interviews, April 8, 10, 1992; Fiedler, 1986).

Race was also an issue raised by some opponents in an effort to divide the community over the SBHC. At public hearings and before the school board, opponents argued that teen pregnancy and sexually related problems were "more of a black than white issue" (Interview, county official, April 8, 1992). "They [meaning blacks] ought not to be having all these babies," claimed one white antagonist (Interview, April 8, 1992). Others cited general statistics on AIDS to suggest that it was a black, not white, problem.

While there were already significant black-white divisions both in the community and on the school board, this tactic was not very successful in exacerbating these divisions. Most white children attended private schools and would not be affected by the clinic. Furthermore, advocates made it clear that clinic funding would not come from local sources and therefore local taxpayers would not be paying for these health services. It was also apparent that the few white youth in the public schools were often as disadvantaged as blacks and therefore extremely needful of basic health services provided by such a clinic. Finally, both whites and blacks desperately wanted to do something to reduce the high rate of welfare among black teenage girls with children, and the SBHC was perceived as a useful approach (Interviews, April 8, 10, 1992).

Despite the determination of Quincy's public officials to protect their SBHC, the Catholic Conference, representing eight dioceses and nearly 2 million Florida parishioners, proved formidable. Contending that the clinic promoted sexual promiscuity and abortion, the Conference convinced Governor Graham to block state financing. Yet other funding was found to keep the health center open (Birk,

1986). However, when the new governor, Robert Martinez (R), took office in 1987, the Catholic Conference renewed its efforts to close the clinic. Martinez was a staunch Catholic and opposed to the provision of contraceptives on school campuses and to unlimited access to abortion. Under pressure from the Conference and other conservative groups, Governor Martinez ordered the Shanks health clinic to move off campus. The governor also attempted to block federal funds to support a SBHC in Miami, but the funds were siphoned through a private organization that then offered health services through the schools. The controversy surrounding these decisions was immense and served to mobilize groups both for and against reproductive services for youth (Emihovich and Herrington, 1997; Interviews, April 8, 10, 1992).

The clinic at Shanks High School was relocated only across the street, but the order to move was significant because it created a new awareness of the political vulnerability of this health service. Moreover, in practical terms, students had to have permission to leave campus in order to walk across the street and use the clinic. With this change, student utilization of the health center declined by more than 30 percent (*Final Report,* 1995).

Despite the turmoil caused by the political controversy and shift in location, the clinic proved to have a great deal of local support and strong leadership. A community advisory council for the health center was established with representation from a variety of groups, including interested citizens, parents, students, teachers, local physicians, ministers, the school board, and clinic staff. Black ministers played a particularly important role because they were the primary form of communication with the African-American community. The advisory council, along with the local Governor's Constituency For Children, provided significant community support for the SBHC, lobbied the school board and state legislature, wrote letters to and spoke with media representatives, and provided feedback to clinic personnel. In addition, experienced, dedicated, and dynamic leaders initiated plans for the clinic and guided its establishment through the first tumultuous years. The school nurse, health department officials, the principal, and the superintendent of schools were key advocates of the health center, demonstrating unusually astute political awareness and skills (*Final Report,* 1995; Interviews, April 8, 10, 1992).

These elements were crucial for the Shanks clinic not only to survive but to thrive in its early years. It was clearly of great value to many disadvantaged students. Independent evaluations showed high utilization rates—66 percent of students during the first year and 73 percent in the second year. Staffed by an advanced nurse practitioner, a part-time nurse, a receptionist, and local physicians who volunteered several hours each week, the health center offered a range of services including health screenings and medical treatment, family planning counseling and contraceptive services, nutrition education, immunizations, abuse counseling, parenting classes, and classroom instruction (Kirby, Waszak, and Zielgler, 1989).

More important, the clinic had highly beneficial effects on student behavior. During the first year of operation, excused absences due to illness dropped by 25 percent and the school dropout rate declined by 21 percent. The most dramatic impact, however, was the significant reduction in teenage pregnancies. In the first two years after the health center opened, teen pregnancies at the school were reduced 75 percent. In addition, following the establishment of the SBHC, the proportion of students who were sexually active remained virtually the same, not increasing as opponents had predicted (Center for Human Services Policy and Administration, 1989). As a result, Quincy's clinic gained a great deal of positive media attention, was visited by state officials, and was praised by one state legislator as a "success story" (Harper, 1989). Well-known 1988 presidential candidate Jesse Jackson appeared at Shanks High School and the health center during his campaign, commending the clinic and advocating the establishment of more SBHCs. This publicity inspired the state legislature to draft and pass the Full Service School Act in 1990. The legislation called for the funding of SBHCs in Florida counties with high teenage pregnancy rates (*Final Report,* 1995; Harper, 1990).

Despite its early success, the Quincy health center continued to be embroiled in political controversy. In 1991, newly elected Governor Lawton Chiles (D), in one of his first official acts, returned the health clinic to its original site inside Shanks High School. Chiles, a strong advocate of increased health care for youth, had praised the Quincy clinic in a statewide televised debate during his campaign (DuPont-Smith, 1991). With this significant political victory, opposition to the health center began to subside. Later in 1991, increased support enabled the clinic to begin expanding into a full service health clinic, adding space and staff to provide more services, particularly mental health care, both for students and their families. The expansion was the result of collaborative efforts by local private organizations, the school district, and the county health department (*Final Report,* 1995). In addition, in 1993 the state legislature, building on the success of the Shanks clinic, allocated funds for two more SBHCs in the county (DuPont-Smith, 1993).

By 1995, however, the state political winds shifted once again. A serious economic recession had greatly reduced state revenues. With a conservative state legislature and increased citizen demands for fighting crime, funding for education and social services was cut significantly. Representatives from populous south Florida now controlled the state legislature, including most leadership positions, and health care monies were increasingly shifted from sparsely populated northern counties to those in the southern part of the state (Colburn and deHaven-Smith, 1999).

In Gadsden County, the health department budget, the primary provider of funds for the Shanks High School clinic, was reduced by 25 percent due to state funding cuts. Over the next three years the Shanks health center's budget suffered cuts in proportion to those of the health department. With no other sources of outside funding, and in a community mired deep in poverty and therefore with no tax resources, the Shanks clinic began to deteriorate. By 1998, its budget was approximately $100,000, the same as its annual allocation in the late 1980s and therefore appreciably less after controlling for rising costs and inflation. Social services and mental health care, the keystone of Shanks' full service center, were cut, along with additional personnel. The clinic's hours were reduced both during the school year and in the summer. A skeleton staff, consisting only of a nurse practitioner and a receptionist, remained, and students were often referred to outside agencies for treatment. Although the level of health care needs among adolescents remained high, only an estimated 23 percent of the students at Shanks actually used the clinic in 1998 (Interviews, December 10, 11, 1998). With the election of Jeb Bush (R) as Governor in 1998, and continued Republican dominance in the legislature, the chances for additional funds for the clinic appear slim.

Local support for the SBHC has ebbed as well. The clinic's community advisory board, once well organized and politically effective, was abandoned due to changes in clinic personnel and funding cuts.

The crisis in teenage pregnancies had been the major mobilizing factor in the 1980s, but with the reductions in pregnancy rates (still one of the highest in the state) and the initiation of other community programs focusing on this issue, the "crisis mentality" subsided. Outside political opposition to the health center, once a rallying cry for local citizens, also faded as birth control dispensation became more common and accepted. Although controversy surrounding the clinic disappeared, so did media, and especially newspaper, coverage that had been so supportive in the 1980s and early 1990s. Many of the dynamic leaders and health center advocates of the past were now gone or their interests had shifted to other priorities. The once high profile and status of the Shanks SBHC had reached its nadir. "Most people here are indifferent to the high school health clinic," stated a respected black leader. "It's there, and parents and students expect it, but if it closed down, it wouldn't inspire a rally to keep it open" (Interview, December 11, 1998). It is a malaise that has led to the decline of many SBHCs.

Jersey City (NJ): An SBHC in Demise

A city well known for its high rate of crime and history of political corruption, Jersey City is one of the poorest, predominantly minority cities in New Jersey. Among its 228,000 residents in 1990, African Americans made up 30 percent and Hispanics some 25 percent, with an overall poverty rate of 19 percent, well above the national average of 13 percent (U.S. Bureau of the Census, 1990). Within Jersey City, Snyder High School is located amid neighborhoods filled with gang violence and drug dealers. Ninety-three percent of Snyder's students are African American, 5 percent Hispanic, and 85 percent qualified for free or reduced lunch programs in 1998. Only about one-third of all students who entered the high school as freshmen graduated. Very high rates of substance abuse, pregnancy, STDs including HIV/AIDS, and various forms of violence, including homicide, characterized the health status of these youth (Leir, 1986a). A 1987 survey of some 1,500 Snyder students and their parents revealed that 450 had health problems they did not know about, and 200 had never visited a doctor. Nurses at the school reported seeing 75 to 100 students a day (Leir, 1987).

It was within this context that the superintendent of schools initiated a proposal for a clinic at Snyder. He approached a member of the school board who had a thorough knowledge of SBHCs and who had worked previously with community organizations and parents. The school board member recruited parents, members of community agencies, school personnel, and health professionals for a planning committee that drafted a proposal to the Robert Wood Johnson Foundation. Letters about the proposal were sent home to parents; public hearings were held; and the media (local newspapers and television) provided important coverage. In the end, school board members, four of whom were minority representatives, passed the proposal by a 6-3 vote (Personal interviews, November 21-22, 1991).

In 1987 Jersey City was one of ten sites in the nation to be awarded a $600,000 grant over four years from RWJ to establish a school-based clinic at Snyder. The sponsoring agent for the SBHC was the Jersey City Medical and Family Health Center, a very supportive resource (Leir, 1987). The Center helped write the proposal and develop the facilities, and ultimately monitored the clinic. The school nurse welcomed the SBHC and became an important referral source for students. In addition, she convinced teachers, who originally were somewhat resistant, that the clinic was a helpful and valuable resource (Personal interviews, clinic personnel, November 21-22, 1991).

Before the arrival of the SBHC at Snyder, however, significant controversy developed over the possible dispensing of contraceptives and information on birth control and abortion. At a public hearing of the State Assembly Education Committee held at city hall in Jersey City early in 1987, proponents and opponents hotly debated these issues. Testimony from representatives of the statewide Catholic Conference, Right to Life organization, Christian Council, and a Republican state legislator were among those strongly opposed to making birth control available to youth. Among those testifying in support of contraceptive accessibility were medical, public health, and local elected officials (Clolery, 1987; Personal interviews, November 21-22, 1991). Even prior to this public conflict, the mayor, the school superintendent, and the school board had argued over the reproductive care issue. The mayor, the most powerful local official and the person who appointed school board members, strongly objected to birth control availability for students. Not surprisingly, the school board decided that no birth control devices would be procured through the

SBHC (Leir, 1986b). They did, however, permit the clinic to provide family planning counseling due to their concern about the high teenage pregnancy rate. Opponents of the Snyder SBHC, most of whom were white, were less tenacious because the student population at Snyder was mostly African American, with a very high teen pregnancy and STD rate (Personal interviews, school officials, November 21-22, 1991).

The clinic opened in 1988 staffed by a full-time counselor and a full-time nurse practitioner who performed general physical exams, treated minor illnesses, and conducted health education workshops. In addition, part-time personnel included a dentist, nutritionist, psychologist, family planning counselor, pediatrician, and an obstetrician-gynecologist. Leslie Morris, appointed clinic director, was a black woman who had previously counseled teens in Baltimore and Boston and had recently earned a master's of public health degree from the University of North Carolina (Dietrich, 1988). Morris proved to have both superior health administrative skills and the ability to develop good rapport with students and with school personnel. She held an open house on parents' night to introduce the clinic. She was also very adept at utilizing the media, and eventually appeared on national television (the *Today* show) with some of her students. Morris made certain that the newspaper covered the clinic in focus pieces. Her efforts impressed all involved with the SBHC. As a teacher and member of the community advisory board claimed, "She's a workaholic, but totally devoted to kids and to their parents. She was a real catalyst behind the clinic opening" (Personal interview, November 21, 1991).

The community advisory board, required by RWJ grant protocols, was composed of a broad cross section of community members, including parents, religious leaders, health agency officials, physicians, students, and representatives from black and Hispanic interest groups such as the local National Association for the Advancement of Colored People (NAACP), Political Association of Spanish-Speaking Organizations (PASSO), and the Urban League. The board met monthly and was important in making the community aware of the health care needs of youth and the functions of the clinic. Likewise, it identified the needs and problems within the community for the clinic personnel. The next several years brought a change in school system personnel, some of whom had been supportive members of the advisory board. Subsequently, the advisory board began to meet less regularly and its importance declined. Despite the disintegration of the board, backing for the clinic remained strong among parents, students, school personnel, the local medical center, black organizations in the community, and local politicians, including the school board (Personal interviews, November 1991).

After a year of operation, the clinic had logged nearly 3,000 visits by 850 students, and had enrolled over 80 percent of students in the school. School attendance, which had been sagging prior to the development of the SBHC, improved. To address a lack of understanding among adolescents about sexuality and STDs, the clinic began pregnancy prevention classes for ninth graders. In addition, the clinic treated a host of acute illnesses, provided required immunizations, offered physical exams, developed classes for handicapped students, trained a number of students in cardiopulmonary resuscitation (CPR), and made a training videotape with students on the lifesaving technique (Leir, 1989). By 1991 the clinic had developed a dropout prevention program which addressed issues ranging from homicide, violence, and drug abuse to self-esteem, career planning, and general life skills. Given the lack of black male representation as health center clients, professional black men were recruited as volunteers to work with male students, and the clinic emphasized services that were attractive to males (i.e., sports physicals, dental screenings, and STD testing). Student visits increased to 4,000 for the 1990-1991 year, with the sharpest increase in patient visits for family planning due to the addition of a full-time OB/GYN nurse practitioner (*Annual Progress Report: Snyder High School,* 1991).

During that period, the state proved to be a strong proponent of school-based health care: the New Jersey Department of Human Services added $6 million to its budget in 1987 to develop health and service programs in schools. In the late 1980s, this was the most substantial effort by any state to link schools and social services to help youth. By 1991 New Jersey was helping to support twenty-nine SBHC programs (Snyder's was not included because it was privately funded), mandating that each center provide core services including mental health and family counseling, drug and alcohol counseling, and general health care. Family planning services were optional, left to local school districts to decide. No state funds, however, could be used to pay for contraceptives or referral for abortion services (Dryfoos, 1994).

In the late 1980s, the state took control of the Jersey City School District due to findings of local political corruption and mismanagement. Although state officials were supportive of the SBHC initially and through the early 1990s, this level of support soon changed markedly. In response to a 1990 New Jersey Supreme Court decision calling for greater equalization of funding among school districts, Governor Jim Florio, a liberal Democrat, pushed the Quality Education Act through the legislature. Designed to increase state funds to lower-class, particularly inner-city, school districts, the Act required a large increase in taxes. Despite the pledge that middle-class districts would also benefit from the school finance plan, New Jersey taxpayers erupted in revolt against the tax increase. State legislators, fearful of the growing backlash, scaled back funding for inner-city schools to provide property tax relief (Reed, 1998).

Race was a major factor in the taxpayer revolt and the reduction in equity funds for largely black city schools. A statewide survey of parents indicated that school finance equalization was viewed in mostly racial, not economic, terms. That is, white parents were far more likely to oppose equalization, and minority (black and Hispanic) parents were very supportive of greater funding for poorer schools, even when socioeconomic status and other variables were held constant (Reed, 1994). This white, middle-class backlash to taxes was also evident in the defeat of Florio and the election of Christine Todd Whitman, a conservative Republican, as governor in 1993.

In spite of repeated demands by the state Supreme Court for greater fairness in school funding, the new governor, who was re-elected in 1997, and the legislature continued to ignore court rulings. State taxes were reduced and inner-city schools, including those in Jersey City, received relatively small equalization increases in state funds ("School Equity in New Jersey," 1996; Pulley, 1997). Although the SBHC at Snyder clearly provided care for poor students, the struggle for state equity funds resulted in no monies for the clinic. Local school and health officials had not planned for nor made successful demands for more funding. When the RWJ funding ended in the early 1990s, the Snyder clinic budget declined dramatically—from $300,000 to $100,000 per year of local school district funding. By the mid-1990s the formerly comprehensive clinic at Snyder was reduced to a bare-bones service provider having lost a dental care assistant, a psychologist, and a physician (Personal interviews, school and clinic personnel, May 19, 1999).

The formerly active community advisory board languished with little outside involvement in clinic affairs. Parents, although generally supportive of the SBHC for necessary health care including family planning for their adolescents, rarely participated in school or clinic functions. Even the local media gave little attention or publicity to Snyder's health center. Only when a group of female students organized an abstinence program did the newspaper feature clinic activity. Although this program was a small part of the total offerings, abstinence-only sexuality education programs were in vogue, and *The New York Times* and NBC's *Today* show deemed this event newsworthy and featured this Snyder program and its director (Nieves, 1997).

The mid-1990s brought a new oversight agency as the medical sponsor for the SBHC, Horizon Health Care. This private nonprofit health care organization soon developed conflicts with the clinic director and other personnel for Horizon's unwillingness to expand services or apply for additional resources. Horizon's administration made decisions without seeking input from or consultation with the clinic director or other school officials. However, because virtually all funding for the clinic was shunted through this local agency, its power was significant. Attempts by Leslie Morris to secure outside grants were not supported by Horizon; and although many students were eligible for Medicaid reimbursements, these were difficult to collect due to lack of agreements with local managed care organizations (Personal interviews, May 19, 1999). In prior years, Medicaid reimbursements had accounted for almost 20 percent of the center's budget. The loss of Medicaid along with RWJ funding caused student visits to the center to plummet from an estimated 5,000 to 900 a year, and the percentage of students enrolled in the clinic steadily declined (Making the Grade, 2000).

At the same time, there was tremendous turnover in the central administration at Snyder High School, with seven different principals in eight years. As a result, consistent school support at this critical level of leadership was lacking. In the community as well, support was floundering for the SBHC. The Catholic Church retained its strong presence in the area and strongly opposed family planning. Even black churches, also important institutions in Jersey City, had some ministers of traditional religious orientation who actively opposed offering reproductive health care at the clinic despite their recognition of the high teen pregnancy and STD rates among black youth. Moreover, some parents feared loss of control over their children's health care and other parents adamantly opposed contraceptive services. Because of this resistance, the school board adhered to its earlier decision to prohibit student access to contraceptives based on its continuing fear of public reaction. The clinic was able to institute HIV/AIDS testing, partly as a result of the increased concern generated by the earlier revelation by basketball star Magic Johnson that he was HIV positive.

Through all this turmoil and change the clinic director declined to become politically involved locally as an advocate for the clinic. In her words, "It's important not to get caught up in politics because it's so corrupt; keep politics out of the process. Besides, it takes too much time, and running this clinic is a full-time job" (Personal interview, May 19, 1999). Morris was concerned about keeping a low profile in the community, believing that this tact would enable the clinic to continue offering services in the way she thought most beneficial for the students without controversy or conflict. However, at a crucial time in its existence, the Snyder clinic lacked the school and community support necessary for its survival (Making the Grade, 2000).

What modest success Snyder's health center experienced was attributed to its dynamic, charismatic director who spent twelve years overseeing its implementation from inception in 1988. Taking a deeply personal approach to helping students, Leslie Morris created a safe place for many poor, mainly black, youths that lived in a violent community. She established support groups of troubled teens to help them cope with death in the family, pregnancy, motherhood, drugs, alcohol, fatherhood, teen violence, and other significant issues in their lives. Called "Mommy Morris" by a number of students, she often took them to lunch, invited them to her home, and took troubled students on recreational field trips (Averett, 1998). One Snyder principal called her "the angel" of the school and Morris considered her work her "ministry" (Personal interviews, May 19, 1999). However, without a pay raise in eight years and with lagging support and funding for the clinic, this highly dedicated and dynamic clinic director resigned in frustration in June 1999 to take a position at the national level.

With the loss of its energetic director, the future of the clinic and of the students at Snyder remains in serious jeopardy. With few on-site services left, students who once used the center increasingly go to the local emergency room. Although the center has not officially closed, Morris recently described it as "totally dead" (Making the Grade, 2000:2). As a community activist acknowledged, "We have high teen pregnancy and high dropout rates. The SBHC has been an oasis here amid the bedlam and chaos. There's a crisis in Kosovo, but there's a crisis here too, yet we simply don't respond" (Personal interview, May 19, 1999).

Virginia Beach (VA): Bastion of Conservatism

Popularly known as a city of tourism and military bases, Virginia Beach has emerged politically as a conservative Republican and Christian Right stronghold. With more than 400,000 residents, it is the largest city in a state that is enamored with its southern tradition. The population of Virginia Beach is largely white (80 percent) and relatively prosperous, with a 1990 median household income of $36,271, the highest of any municipality in the commonwealth (U.S. Bureau of the Census, 1990).

Since the late 1980s, Virginia Beach politics has increasingly been dominated by the right wing of the Republican Party. The GOP worked vigorously at the grass roots to mobilize voters and recruit good candidates for local office. The greatest infusion of energy and resources for the party came from the Christian Right, particularly the Christian Coalition. With its home base in Virginia Beach, the Christian Coalition, with almost 2 million members and followers nationwide by the mid-1990s, soon became one of the largest and best organized groups of the Christian Right. Led by Pat Robertson, a Baptist minister, wealthy business mogul, and political activist, the Christian Coalition quickly gained control of the Republican Party in Virginia Beach and in much of the rest of the state as well (Rozell and Wilcox, 1996; Wilcox, 1996).

A sizeable military presence also contributed to the city's conservatism. With four military bases in the area, 57 percent of adult men in Virginia Beach were either actively serving or were veterans of the armed forces in 1990 (U.S. Bureau of the Census, 1990). Active military personnel, however, were relatively mobile and therefore less in-

volved in community politics than other residents. Moreover, the traditional orientation of the military translated into a more moderate
form of political conservatism compared to the city's right-wing religious forces.

Given the nature of the political environment, discussions of establishing school health centers consistently confronted strong, organized opposition. Yet the need for increased health care, especially
reproductive services, for adolescents was evident to a number of Virginia Beach's leaders and health professionals. In 1984, the city was
identified as having one of the highest teen pregnancy rates in the
state (Regan, 1986). STD rates were also high and drug problems
among adolescents were becoming an important issue as well. Pockets
of poverty existed in an otherwise upper middle-class city as the
small black, Asian, and Hispanic populations began to grow, presenting their own special health needs associated with disadvantaged
youth (Interviews, March 9, 11, 1992).

In 1986 representatives from local public and private organizations
began meeting to discuss programs to prevent teenage pregnancies.
Calling the area's rate of adolescent pregnancy "near epidemic," the
twenty-five member committee represented school personnel, public
health officials, and representatives from social service, family
service, and mental health agencies in Virginia Beach and nearby
Norfolk. The Junior League (a women's organization), the school
systems of both cities, and a nonprofit areawide agency for human
services called the Planning Council developed the committee in a
quiet manner. One plan of pregnancy prevention studied by the group
was the concept of comprehensive health clinics at schools that
would provide students ready access to sexuality education and counseling. A planning task force researched such programs at thirty-one
schools in eighteen cities across the nation. They found that the
SBHCs that provided sex education and contraceptives or birth control prescriptions helped to reduce teen pregnancies and school dropouts. The committee accepted the idea of looking further into the pos-
sibility of establishing school-based clinics in Norfolk and Virginia
Beach, and proposed a $7,500 planning grant from the city councils
of each municipality (Regan, 1986).

The Norfolk City Council quickly passed the proposal and began
to make plans for the establishment of a school health center. In Virginia Beach, however, the proposal immediately attracted formidable

opposition from several religious groups and parents. Prior to a public hearing on the city budget, which included the $7,500 request, opponents began to mobilize. Leaflets were distributed at local churches urging members to protest the funding. Many opponents called or sent letters to city council members. At the Virginia Beach budget hearing in April 1986, more than 100 angry citizens turned what is normally a routine meeting into a rally against "sex clinics" in public schools. Although the $7,500 planning proposal was a small part of the city's overall proposed $423 million budget, it dominated the budget hearing. Public speakers at the meeting opposed the planning grant, contending that SBHCs "are harmful to children and society," "promote free and easy promiscuity without guilt," and "don't teach values to uphold the family structure" (Davis, 1986b:D1). The well-organized opponents included representatives of the Christian Coalition, the Rock Church and other fundamentalist Christian churches, the Catholic Church, the Eagle Forum, and the local chapter of the Virginia Society for Human Life, an antiabortion organization (Interviews, March 9, 11, 1992).

The city council was shocked by the number and vehemence of those who attended and spoke at the hearing. "It was the worst night of my life," claimed one city official (Interview, March 9, 1992). Although some advocates of the SBHC planning grant attended the meeting, not one spoke publicly in favor of the funding. Proponents were intimidated by the large, vociferous opposition and were not organized or prepared to deal with such a political outburst. Not surprisingly, the city council voted unanimously in opposition to the planning grant; no council member spoke in favor of the funding. In the words of the mayor of Virginia Beach, "It is a social issue period. It doesn't belong in the schools" (Davis, 1986a:D1). Shortly thereafter, the school board, which had planned to discuss the health clinic proposal in a separate public meeting, canceled such plans and abandoned all efforts even to consider a SBHC.

Foreshadowing this SBHC proposal rejection was the Virginia Beach experience with sex education, one of the most controversial issues in the city's schools. In the 1970s, when sex education first became a political issue, significant conflict occurred between those who favored such education in the public schools and those who opposed it. Caught between these forces were Virginia Beach's public schools, which had no mandate from the state or from parents to teach about human sexuality. Statewide, only fifty of 137 school districts had some form of sex education. Many school boards, including the board for Virginia Beach, lacked a clear community consensus and therefore did not even discuss sexuality education programs. Indeed, early advocates of sex education met with strong, vocal opposition. In 1982, opponents sponsored a conference in Virginia Beach featuring a nationally prominent foe of sex education who spoke of destroying a child's "holy bashfulness" and "natural shame" by prematurely mentioning sex. Sponsoring organizations included local Catholic churches, the Eagle Forum, the American Life Lobby, and Citizens Against Unacceptable Sex Education (Laws, 1986).

In contrast to Virginia Beach, plans for a school-based health center in Norfolk moved ahead relatively smoothly. A clinic planning committee was organized and involved elements of the larger community, including representatives of churches, the PTA, student groups, the health department, school officials, the school board, and the city council. The committee held public meetings to educate local citizens, emphasizing that the proposed clinic would provide comprehensive health care and encourage postponement of sexual activity, thus avoiding harmful consequences. The committee also initiated media coverage to promote these clinic goals. Many of those on the planning committee ultimately served on the clinic advisory board, which was established prior to the opening of the SBHC to build and maintain community support. The Norfolk clinic, the first in the state, was instituted in 1987 at Lake Taylor High School, the majority of whose students were African-American low-income youth (Mayfield, 1986).

Due to the extensive planning, publicity, and public education, there was little active opposition to the Norfolk school clinic. Lack of resistance also was attributed to the documented high teen pregnancy rate and high levels of other health care needs of students at the Lake Taylor site. In addition, because a private donor provided the initial funds for this clinic, no school or city money needed to be allocated. In a community that is more moderate politically than Virginia Beach, even most church groups in Norfolk were either supportive or at least not openly opposed to the SBHC. Much of the relatively large black population mobilized in support because these black adolescents had significant unmet health care needs. Nonetheless, a number of active opponents from Virginia Beach emerged because they feared that if a clinic opened in Norfolk it would pave the way for SBHCs in their own city. Whenever a public meeting about the proposed Norfolk clinic took place, several Virginia Beach citizens would picket in protest. In the end, the approval of the Norfolk school health center was contingent on stipulations that parental consent would be required, that no birth control would be available on site, and that there would be no mention of abortion by clinic staff (Interviews, March 9, 11, 1992; Regan, 1987).

Not long after the major conflict over SBHCs in Virginia Beach, debate erupted in 1987 over a state mandated Family Life Education curriculum that was proposed by the state board of education. A major portion of this curriculum focused on sex education. As in previous discussions of sex education and more recently of school health centers, adversaries were numerous and outspoken. Even before the curriculum was passed by the Virginia General Assembly, dozens of angry parents appeared at local school board meetings to register their complaints. Although the sex education proposal allowed parents to excuse their children from such classes and gave localities a degree of autonomy in teaching the curriculum, many parents expressed concern about these and other issues. Some feared that schools would be usurping the authority of parents, and others objected to the proposed instruction about birth control instead of teaching only about abstinence until marriage. Very few persons testified in favor of the curriculum (Sussman, 1987).

Family Life Education was ultimately adopted by the state, but local opposition to mandated sex education grew in size and intensity. Religious groups in particular organized to influence the nature of what would be taught n Virginia Beach schools. Aligned with these groups was the Family Foundation, a conservative statewide organization affiliated with Focus on the Family, and the local chapter of Concerned Women of America, which soon became one of the most powerful right-wing organizations in the state (Rozell and Wilcox, 1996). Discussions about birth control were eliminated and greater emphasis was placed on parents as primary sex educators. In essence, the local school board succumbed to the tremendous political pressure of conservative groups and "watered down the curriculum substantially" (Interview, city official, March 11, 1992). So powerful was the opposition that the only two strong school board proponents of the state sex education program were soon replaced with more conservative members by the city council.

In the minds of many Virginia Beach residents, the issues of school health clinics and sex education were inextricably linked. Both raised fundamental questions concerning teenage sexuality, pregnancy, and parental versus school responsibility. The mass mobilization of conservatives, particularly traditional religious organizations, enabled them to control local politics on these basic issues. Moreover these early political victories had long-term consequences. According to a school board member, "The success of the opposition created a more conservative approach to controversial issues in dealing with societal problems" (Interview, March 9, 1992). Other Virginia Beach officials concurred. "Now it's difficult to get any program discussed or passed to deal with teen pregnancy . . . even though the school administration has changed a few times since 1986, there is an 'institutional memory'" (Interview, city official, March 9, 1992).

Other factors bolstered the dominance of conservatives. In 1993 the school district switched to an elected, rather than appointed, school board. The change occurred as a result of right-wing pressure, and it enabled well-mobilized religious and other conservative groups to increasingly control the political makeup of the board. In addition, local Republicans, assisted by the Christian Coalition, increased their numbers and grassroots organization in the 1990s, becoming a large majority of the voting public and electing Virginia Beach officials and state representatives by ever-increasing margins. The demographic influx of Republicans statewide altered Virginia politics as well, with the GOP gaining control of both houses of the legislature and the governorship by the late 1990s (Interview, Virginia Beach supervisor of elections, July 11, 2000). Clearly the city and the state have shifted to the political right, with greater emphasis on fiscal and social conservatism (Rozell and Wilcox, 1996).

Not surprisingly given the political environment, there were no serious attempts to reintroduce the idea of SBHCs in Virginia Beach. Fear of the active opposition persuaded advocates to give up discussions of school health clinics. Moreover, due to budget cuts in education by Republicans at both the state and local levels, funds for new services were no longer available. With a nurse in every school and the presence of a public health department, most local officials perceived health care for youth as adequate. In a primarily middle-class city with few minorities, most families were medically insured and had their own doctors. Military personnel and their children received free medical care (Interviews, May 27-29, 1998). Furthermore, teen pregnancy rates declined significantly in the 1990s, with rates in Virginia Beach dropping more precipitously than those statewide (King, 1998). Large numbers of adolescent pregnancies had been one of the potent factors in initiating discussions of SBHCs in the city.

Despite its prosperity, Virginia Beach has a sizable and growing number of children and adolescents with health care needs. The percentage of minority (mostly African-American) students rose from 22 percent in 1988 to 34 percent by 1998. The number of students receiving free or reduced lunches, an indicator of poverty, more than doubled between 1987 and 1997, reaching 26 percent in the latter year (*School Division Facts,* 1997). In terms of health care, school nurses typically provide minimal primary care for an average of 1,200 students per nurse. Because of budget cuts, the local public health department was reduced in 1998 from four sites to one for serving youth. Many students are not aware of the poorly publicized health department services. Youth have also found the service sites inaccessible because of the distance from their schools and homes and the city's inadequate public transportation. As a result, relatively few adolescents have used the only public health service that offers reproductive care and drug abuse and mental health services (Interviews, health care providers, May 27-29, 1998).

In terms of primary prevention of reproductive health problems, the increasingly conservative state government voted in 1998 to make Family Life Education a matter of local prerogative. Previously this sexuality education curriculum was mandated by the state, but with a good deal of local autonomy about what was taught and the grade levels in which the instruction was offered. Parents always had the option of keeping their children out of such classes (Editorial, 1998). The new law had little effect in Virginia Beach schools, simply reinforcing the local control of sex education that had already diluted the curriculum to one of the most conservative in the state. Controversial topics such as birth control, STDs, and homosexuality were not addressed, and other issues could be discussed only at certain grade levels regardless of whether students were ready and/or wanted the information before that time. As one high-level school official summarized it, "Abstinence-only based curriculum is the tack that is taken, and not much is discussed until grades nine and ten. Students are told to 'go ask their parents' about sex" (Interview, May 28, 1998).

In spite of the political atmosphere, some health and education professionals attempted to address the health needs of youth in a more comprehensive manner. In 1996, the School Health Initiative for Education, a coalition of school nurses, medical personnel, and parents, was established to promote the physical and mental health of youth. Similarly, a school health advisory board, representing students, teachers, parents, and other elements of the community, was initiated in 1991. Both organizations studied and issued reports on concerns such as staffing of school nurses, student health informational systems, and school safety. Neither organization, however, discussed or recommended programs to deal with reproductive health care, alcohol or drug abuse, school violence, or other potentially controversial but important problems of youth. Better Beginnings Coalition, a small peer-mentoring program for teenagers established in 1995, helps to provide accurate information for high-risk students. Even though this initiative emphasizes sexuality issues, it is limited to only a few schools and by its abstinence-only approach (Dooley, 1998; Interview, health professional, May 29, 1998).

School-based health clinics are no longer discussed in Virginia Beach. Yet city officials claim that many parents want more comprehensive sexuality education and would not oppose the consideration of SBHCs. Nonetheless officials concede that the conservative political climate does not permit this. "If we brought it [SBHC] up, it wouldn't get off the ground," contended one health official. "It's still a politically loaded topic . . . very emotionally charged. People in the schools are deterred from discussion of it. We run into difficulties with anything to do with sex. Some think schools should stay out of family life" (Interview, May 27, 1998).

Although the opposition may be a "vocal minority," they are extremely well organized, have resources, and are politically astute. None of these things are true for advocates of a more comprehensive health care and sexuality education curriculum for youth. Furthermore, the state political atmosphere is unfriendly to the concept of school health centers. In 1998, Virginia reported only twelve SBHCs, one of the lowest totals of any state similar in student size. The state allocates no funds to directly support such clinics, and provides little nonfinancial assistance (Making the Grade, 1998). One state official from Virginia Beach summarized the view of many Virginians:

> Schools should not be providing birth control, condoms, or abortion referrals. Schools should focus on what is their basic charter, teaching reading, writing, and math. Having government take these [health care] roles reinforces the breakdown of the family. Government takes the burden from parents, but doesn't do it well, and the family in turn takes less responsibility." (Interview, May 27, 1998)

This is the prevailing political philosophy in a locale that has virtually banned school health centers.

Chapter 3

The Establishment and Success of School Health Reforms

The clinic has had many benefits. All the young women who were pregnant have finished school, as opposed to dropping out and not completing high school. Other health problems have been identified through the SBHC; for example, heart defects, potential suicides, and physical abuse. The clinic provides, for many, the first physical examination they have had in their lives. Attendance and grades of students have increased. I am very pleased and proud of the results of this pioneering, risky venture.

Interview, school administrator, rural Florida community

In many cities and states across the country there is a growing consensus that changes and improvements in health care are needed for children and adolescents, especially those from poor families. One significant innovation that has proved helpful in meeting this need is the school-based health clinic model. Yet general consensus alone is not sufficient to establish and maintain such clinics. The efforts to bring about this reform involve the politics of social change. The process of politics is abhorred by many as inherently dirty and corrupt, and certainly confusing and difficult to understand. Educators in particular hold these views, and believe that the world of education is somewhat separate from the world of politics. As we have mentioned, these perceptions are beginning to change as schools consider and initiate programs of reform (Wirt and Kirst, 1989).

Instituting school reform, such as SBHCs, directly involves the politics of making structural changes in the educational system. Such changes affect school governance and personnel, school relations with the larger community and even the state government, and the integration of health services into the overall educational program. Each of these changes is important in the process of establishing and sustaining school clinics. Scholars of school reform have found that educational changes are most likely to occur when supported by a broad-based political coalition of education groups, parents and their associations, students, community activists, the media, business leaders, foundations, and other important local leaders and organizations (Gittell, 1994; Orr, 1996; Stone, 1998). Thus reform includes the involvement of local stakeholders beyond school officials and professional educators. Moreover, it is the strength and consistency of this political coalition that is an important determinant of success (Gittell, 1994).

What local groups are typically most crucial to the development of an effective coalition? Obviously teachers and school administrators are key educational stakeholders; schooling is their profession and they most clearly have a vested interest in potential educational change. Local public officials—especially school board members, the school superintendent, and, in many large cities, mayors—also play important roles in school reform. These public officials are critical in making authoritative decisions that either enhance or block changes in schools. An effective alliance must include parents and adolescent students. It is impossible to implement major school reform without the active participation of those likely to be most affected (Orr, 1996).

Beyond groups that are most clearly self-interested in educational change, there are independent community organizations that are often key constituents of reform coalitions. These organizations typically include churches, labor unions, businesses, minority interest groups, nonprofit advocacy groups, universities, and foundations. Often little attention is given to foundations, but in the case of school health clinics and other school reforms they are frequently an invaluable catalyst for change. In addition, business leaders have commonly been an untapped but potentially significant source of support for reform. As employers, businesses have a direct concern in the quality of education of the labor pool. Many also develop a sense of civic responsibility, partly as a matter of good public relations, and are therefore supportive of school and community reforms that promise to promote general welfare (Orr, 1996; Stone, 1998). Finally, successful political coalitions involve at least some major actors at the state level including the governor, members of the legislature, and leaders in the department of education. The state is responsible for contributing almost half of local school funding as well as developing or promoting programs that facilitate educational innovation (Dye, 2000).

Because school districts are limited in their capacity to carry out major reforms alone, school officials must form broad political alliances, or "regimes," with nongovernmental groups to enhance their limited financial and decision-making powers. It is the role of local leaders to build and then to *maintain* effective coalitions for school reform to take place successfully. This ability to form and sustain broad-based alliances is called "civic capacity," and involves two elements. One is participation, meaning that each group in the coalition actually contributes in some way toward the reform. The other element is understanding an issue as a community problem, one that goes beyond individual interests, and therefore calls for a collective or civic response (Stone, 1998). In the case of school-based health centers, civic capacity refers to community groups and individuals forming an enduring coalition with a shared responsibility to act on a common concern—the need for accessible health care by large numbers of youth.

INNER CIRCLE OF SUPPORT

School district officials and personnel comprise the inner circle of support critical to the successful implementation and sustenance of school-based health centers. From the inception, officials at the highest levels, the superintendent and the school board, must be involved as equal partners with the community agency representatives sponsoring the SBHC. These officials' approval and endorsement of SBHC incorporation into the school system is critical for principals to feel sufficiently reinforced for instituting the necessary changes for SBHC integration into their school (Elders, 1993).

Although the support of higher level officials is important, even more crucial is the school principal. As documented in our national survey of clinic directors, fully 93 percent of respondents identified school administrators as strong supporters of their centers; the only source of support rated higher was that of students (see Table 3.1). According to former U.S. Surgeon General Joycelyn Elders (1993),

TABLE 3.1. Perceived Level of Support for SBHCs from School Groups During Last Three Years*

Group	None	Low	Medium	High
Students	0	2	16	82
Administrators	1	6	19	74
Guidance counselors	3	7	21	69
School nurses	9	7	17	68
Teachers	0	6	31	63
Parent organizations	15	8	34	43
School board members	12	14	34	40

*Based on national survey of SBHC directors (N = 226); numbers represent percentages of respondents.

principals, in their powerful role and ultimate responsibility for all functions within the school, are key to effectively planning, implementing, maintaining, and sustaining centers. They perform several important functions in this regard. Principals are primary advocates and promoters for collaboration between school personnel and the community and families. They establish policy regarding how and when clinic appointments may be scheduled for students. Principals can also organize teams of staff to discuss and cooperate in handling individual cases involving students and their families. As Joy Dryfoos (1994) concluded, clinic staff know that they have been fully accepted and integrated when the principal claims ownership of the SBHC (even though the funding typically does not come from the school budget). An ongoing and important challenge for clinic coordinators is to maintain good relations with the principal (and superintendent) because of the high turnover rate in these administrative positions. Generally, principals' support is strong because they appreciate that clinic staff provide substantial relief to their teachers through managing the health needs of students (Allensworth et al., 1997).

Teachers also are essential clinic supporters—two of three clinic directors in our study rated their support at the highest level. Teachers are in a primary position to be influential clinic promoters; they can advocate clinic use to parents, encourage and refer students for clinic services, administer permission slips and surveys, and attend case conferences. Although school policy may be in place to facilitate students' use of the clinic, teachers must cooperate in the process. Some teachers must be convinced of the usefulness and benefits of SBHCs—some are skeptical, believing that sometimes students escape their classes through clinic attendance, while others are resistant due to the belief that schools should not take on the family-based responsibility of health care for youth. A good way for clinic and teaching personnel to meet and understand each other, and their respective roles in health care promotion, is through in-service training programs, particularly concerning psychosocial development of youth. Sometimes clinic staff can garner teacher support by providing limited medical services for school personnel, such as screenings and immunizations. Staff can also volunteer their services to assist teachers in the classroom as guest speakers in science, health, and sex education (Dryfoos, 1994).

Other school staff are necessary for support as well, particularly school nurses and guidance counselors. Some of these professionals may be resistant to outside agencies entering the school because they perceive that instituting an SBHC is an inherent criticism of the care they have been providing for "their" students. Potential antipathy may also be caused by the disparity in professional roles and compensation between school and community-based professionals. School nurses, for instance, are typically paid less than nurse practitioners and have less authority to provide medical care. The issue of confidentiality is yet another area of potential conflict. One of the guiding principles of SBHCs, and a key to their effectiveness in reaching adolescents, is the commitment to maintaining the privacy of youth health concerns. Clinic staff may receive information that school personnel would deem pertinent and that staff cannot share, such as revelations of parental sexual abuse or identification of drug dealers (Dryfoos, 1991).

As demonstrated in our survey, successful programs build bridges with key school personnel. School counselors and nurses were reported as supportive by at least 85 percent of our clinic directors. SBHC sponsors must collaborate with these and other appropriate school-based personnel (such as athletic coaches) in the planning process from the outset and develop procedures that enhance the existing services these school professionals offer. Typically this extensive, multilayered planning effort involves at least a year of preparation, negotiation, and orientation (Dryfoos, 1991; Hacker and Wessel, 1998).

Most parents have been found to be supportive of SBHCs, including in some cases clinical provision of reproductive care services (Emihovich and Herrington, 1997; Santelli et al., 1992; Weathersby, Lobo, and Williamson, 1995). Parents are particularly helpful in obtaining and sustaining widespread community support for centers (Rienzo and Button, 1993; Walter et al., 1995). An effective technique for documenting their support is by conducting parent surveys. Having parent representatives on the SBHC advisory board keeps this crucial source of support informed and active. Parental involvement has proved to be especially beneficial for those SBHCs that have faced some opposition, often from citizens who do not have children in the schools in which the centers are established. The prevailing practice of SBHCs requiring signed parental consent for youth to use the clinic creates additional evidence of this support. Very few parents in schools with clinics refuse to allow their children access to clinic services. Our survey reported that an average of 67 percent of students were enrolled in SBHCs with parental permission. Most times the consent form is "all or none" in terms of service provision (Rienzo and Button, 1993; Emihovich and Herrington, 1997).

Finally, it is imperative that SBHCs have the support of their clientele, students. Of course, student support ultimately is demonstrated by their actions—whether and to what extent they solicit the services offered by clinics. In that regard, planners can be confident. Numerous studies show that students, especially those in most need, highly value and use the variety of services their SBHCs offer. In one of the only empirical studies of student attitudes, Santelli, Kouzis, and Newcomer (1996) confirmed their overwhelming support, and found that the major influences on the positive feelings of students were their peers and their own experiences with clinics. Julia Graham Lear, director of the Robert Wood Johnson Foundation national support program for SBHCs, "Making the Grade," explains that the key component of student support is the clinic personnel:

> School-based health centers have staff who really love kids, and the teenagers pick up on that. That is what makes the centers such a terrific resource. They encourage kids to come, which is

the toughest part, because if the kids don't want to come in, you can't help them. (Howley, 2000:B5)

OUTER CIRCLE OF SUPPORT

The success of school health clinics is crucially dependent upon support and alliances with a host of organizations and governmental structures beyond the confines of the school system. As early as 1988 Philip Porter, director of the School-Based Adolescent Health Care Program, claimed, "I don't know a successful clinic that doesn't have a parent or community organization behind it" (Making the Grade, 1998:4). Ten years later, Julia Graham Lear argued that outside collaboration was more important than ever. "With no obvious or certain means of long-term funding, school-based health centers need to make their case to the community," she claimed (Making the Grade, 1998:4). Today, successful clinics have developed relationships with a variety of organizations ranging from private foundations, various levels of government, and health care institutions to community professional organizations, churches, businesses, social services, and organizations of parents.

Developing this outer circle of support is essential to SBHCs. In the early stages of clinic development, the most important benefits are increased resources and gaining greater acceptance in the community. Resources, especially funding, are the lifeblood of SBHCs and are especially vital to long-term viability. Beyond these basic advantages, school health clinic relationships with community and other organizations often provide the clinic with an enhanced image in the community, increased access to services and to other populations, and greater advocacy efforts on behalf of the clinic. Moreover, in the process of developing partnerships, clinics and other organizations may identify common ground on which to collaborate further in improving health care for youth and other citizens in the community. In return, partners with SBHCs experience a sense of altruism, provide a public service, and give something back to the community in which they function (Juszczak, Moody, and Vega-Matos, 1998).

Relationships between school health clinics and organizations can take a variety of forms, including networking, coordination, collaboration, and formal contractual agreements for funds or services. The most important organizational issue for SBHCs is identification of a "lead" outside agency and the kind of collaborative plan that is forged with this agency. Although these health clinics are located within schools, more than 90 percent of SBHCs are administered and funded by outside lead organizations. Community health and social service agencies are the most common of these agencies, but their relationships with school clinics may take any of the forms mentioned.

Few school systems are capable of taking on the entire responsibility for delivering comprehensive health and social services to students. Moreover teachers and school administrators prefer to concentrate on academic concerns. Sponsorship of SBHCs by outside agencies has other advantages as well. Funding is the major benefit, since community organizations are eligible for and have access to a variety of public and private funding sources. They also facilitate access to third-party reimbursements, particularly Medicaid. In addition, outside sponsorship eliminates the need for school medical liability insurance, facilitates student referrals to and entry into community agencies, and provides another significant advocate for school health centers (Dryfoos, 1994; Fox, Wicks, and Lipson, 1992).

Beyond lead agencies that are absolutely critical to their success, SBHCs have attained support from relatively few community organizations. In our national survey of clinic directors, we asked about the level of support provided to school clinics by community groups outside the school system. Table 3.2 summarizes the results. The groups judged as providing the most support are social service and health care agencies. These are typically lead agencies that often sponsor SBHCs. If not directly sponsoring the school clinics, they have a clear and direct interest in helping to provide basic services to youth through the schools and through accepting student referrals from SBHCs. Various parent organizations are also quite supportive, according to clinic directors. Parents have a vested interest in school clinics that help meet the health needs of their children. Other than these organizations, however, no other community groups offer much support, mainly because they are rarely solicited for help.

Physicians and businesses are two of the most prominent, politically important, and resource-rich groups in most communities. Yet SBHCs have obtained very little support from these potentially helpful sources (see Table 3.2). For other organizations, a vested interest in SBHCs is not as clear, and much time and effort must be expended to attempt to build recognition and support of school clinics. A major

TABLE 3.2. Perceived Level of Support for SBHCs from Community Groups During Last Three Years*

Group	None	Low	Medium	High
Social service organizations	18	7	28	47
Health care agencies	11	9	34	45
Parent organizations	20	16	30	34
Youth organizations	36	18	25	21
Private physicians	31	29	28	12
Business leaders	43	18	28	12
Churches	47	22	22	9

*Based on national survey of SBHC directors (N = 226); numbers represent percentages of respondents.

reason for this lack of support is that few clinic directors recognize the significance of building community support beyond agencies that would have a clear and direct interest in SBHCs. In the words of a longtime clinic director in a Denver (CO) high school, "I did not appreciate it previously, but building political support in the community is very important." Other experienced directors echoed this sentiment. Indeed, in listing factors that contributed most to SBHC success, clinic heads mentioned "community support" second most frequently in our national survey.

The establishment of community advisory boards enhances the process of building community support for SBHCs. Such boards are typically inclusive, representing a broad range of community organizations. Parents, school officials, students, and health and social services are the primary groups represented and those with the most direct concerns about school health clinics. Broader representation, however, was found on many advisory boards that included school board and other public officials, business leaders, ministers, civic leaders, and opponents of SBHCs. Foundations and other funding agencies often required some form of advisory group to guide the grassroots planning effort. Yet even after the initial process of planning, advisory boards have proved helpful in building community support, increasing public awareness, identifying future leaders and funding sources, and managing controversy (Ridini, 1998; Santelli, Morreale, et al., 1996).

Surprisingly, few studies have explored the role of community advisory boards in the long-term success of school clinics. Although these boards have been utilized during the planning stages, there is little knowledge about whether SBHCs have maintained their advisory organizations and, if so, what functions they have provided. Our national surveys in 1991 and 1998 both attest to the importance of community advisory groups. The 1991 survey found that 80 percent of SBHCs (many of them in their initial stages of development) had advisory boards, that the boards were large in number (averaging seventeen members) and relatively inclusive of community organizations. We concluded that the boards were "crucial for creating and maintaining community support," and that they also served to advise staff, monitor programs, and provide advocacy (Rienzo, 1994).

Seven years later the results of our second national survey indicated that fewer school clinics had maintained their advisory organizations and those that did so had boards that were smaller. About two-thirds (65 percent) of SBHCs reported having some form of advisory group, and the average membership numbered eight. Providing community outreach and greater acceptance of SBHCs are useful functions, but clearly advisory boards are no longer as important as they were during the formative stages of clinic development. By 1998, only 5 percent of clinic directors mentioned their community advisory boards as factors that contribute to the maintenance and growth of their health center. Although maintaining an advisory board no longer seems as important to the success of SBHCs, further analysis of the data showed that student usage of clinic services was positively associated with greater inclusiveness of advisory board membership (Rienzo, Button, and Wald, 2000).

BUILDING THE WEB OF SUPPORT

A "coordinator of planning" or clinic director generally holds the responsibility for generating and sustaining these inner and outer circles that comprise the fundamental sources of support for SBHCs. As documented in our earlier national study of the establishment of SBHCs (Rienzo, 1994), the characteristics most highly associated with clinic success were the ability of coordinators to enthusiastically communicate about and to secure funding for their clinics, and the willingness to commit substantial time to planning efforts. Their expertise in adolescent health care (i.e., coordinators are health care providers) was the sole characteristic predictive of the capacity of clinics to offer reproductive health care services. In general, clinic directors should be strong leaders with a passion for the welfare of youth and the skills to coordinate various services and to establish support (Dryfoos, 1994). Comments elicited when directors in our 1998 survey were asked to identify the most important factors that contributed to their clinic success reinforced these claims. Virtually every comment reflected the need to build solid support within the school and the community. As a respondent from Arizona stated, "[The head of the] Family Resource and Wellness Program in the district wrote the grant for start up, garnered support of key administrators in schools and school board members, served as a strong advocate for the program, and developed liaisons with community health center providing services." Another fundamental component of building and maintaining this web of support is the ability to work with and through the media.

ROLE OF THE MEDIA

The media—newspapers, radio, and television—perform two important roles in communities. First of all, they are public informers, making sure that important information is available to citizens. Second, some media, especially newspapers, also assume the role of influencing the direction of public opinion and public policy. These roles may overlap, of course, as providing or not providing information or deciding in what manner to present information can be a way of influencing people (Kweit and Kweit, 1999).

There are limits on the ability of the media to cover local political issues. Typically few resources are devoted to covering local politics because such news coverage is considered uninteresting to readers. Most Americans are more attracted to stories concerning national political affairs so the media cover local issues in a restricted way and primarily as a civic duty. As a result of low citizen interest and sparse media coverage, there is a tendency for news reporters to "substitute glitz and sensation for substance, even when reporting about governmental issues" (Kaniss, 1995:371). This is especially true for local television news, which tends to focus on the scandalous and sensational.

So what do these insights about the media and local politics mean for SBHCs? They strongly suggest the importance of media coverage, and positive portrayals in particular of school health centers and their activities. In terms of creating positive or negative public images, of informing and influencing public opinion, and of helping to set the political agenda, the media play a crucial role for many SBHCs. In the planning, initiation, and maintenance of school health centers, publicity generated by the media is a major factor in informing and educating citizens as well as community leaders. These groups and individuals in turn influence public policy, in this case the implementation and sustenance of school clinics.

To utilize the media successfully in this manner, however, depends on who maintains control of the local media. Of course, news editors and media owners have their biases about what is newsworthy, and they have a great deal of power over what is printed or televised. Yet individuals and interest groups with influence or status also have an advantage in acquiring favorable media attention (Graber, 1984). In the case of SBHCs, school superintendents and principals, school board members, well-known physicians, local politicians, health agency professionals, and others who are respected locally must be mobilized as clinic advocates and spokespersons for the media. SBHCs have a natural advantage with news reporters because clinics contribute to community improvement by providing new health care services to children and adolescents. This appeals to media personnel who generally view themselves as "protectors and defenders of the public good" (Kweit and Kweit, 1999:117). This message needs to be emphasized by SBHC advocates with status and power in the community, since there are often competing groups and individuals with negative views of SBHCs.

Opponents of school clinics typically focus on reproductive health care issues, appealing to citizens' fears that clinics encourage sexual activity and even abortion among youth. These controversial claims attract the media because they produce stories that are sensational or dramatic, thus fulfilling the need to generate citizen interest in otherwise mundane local news. With competition for the attention of the media in terms of whose message is favored, SBHC advocates need to be ever mindful and skillful in how to publicize their case, and how to best respond to opponents in the continuing battle over media support.

Results from our two national surveys of SBHCs clearly indicate the importance of media relations in boosting clinic success. In each survey, analysis showed that the greater the number of ways clinic or school personnel communicated through media representatives, the larger the SBHC budget and number of services offered. These findings were true even when controlling for other factors that might be important for clinic success, such as size of school, wealth of the community, or health care needs of students (Rienzo, 1994; Rienzo, Button, and Wald, 2000). Our case studies of SBHCs reinforced these findings. In interviews, proponents of school clinics cited proactive involvement with the media as an important strategy for developing and maintaining health centers (Rienzo and Button, 1993). They specified that initiating contact with the media and publicizing reports about youth health issues, school clinics, and health services provided were very helpful approaches. Proponents also claimed that public relations skills and public relations organizations within the city or school administration were especially useful in gaining timely publicity supportive of SBHCs. In the words of a clinic coordinator in New Mexico, "The media comes out for special events, like a health fair, but not much else. It helps to make clinic news available through the school district and university public relations office" (Interview, May 3, 1999).

Competition with clinic opponents for media attention creates a difficult dilemma for SBHC advocates. To advertise or publicize school health centers and their benefits to the press also risks drawing attention unnecessarily to information about reproductive health care or other potentially controversial services. This kind of information provides the grist for news stories that are sensational because they generate debate, and opponents leap at the opportunity to distort such knowledge to create fear and suspicion about clinic activities (Rienzo and Button, 1993). As a result, many clinic directors avoid publicity and media attention altogether. Our 1998 survey indicated that slightly more than half (54 percent) of SBHC administrators had issued press releases about clinic activities, and only 23 percent reported ongoing communication with news reporters. In addition, barely a majority (57 percent) thought that the media portrayed fairly the functions of their clinic. According to a clinic coordinator in Albuquerque (NM) who believed that media coverage was a key to keeping the public informed about SBHC activities, "I'm leery, however, of being in the media because of family planning issues and the media may just focus on this" (Interview, May 3, 1999). A New York City clinic director who had experienced significant negative repercussions from press attention claimed, "The media portrays the SBHC as people that only give out condoms and birth control pills" (1998 survey response).

The ultimate lesson is that advocates of school health centers need to utilize the media to inform the public and as a way of helping to mobilize support. Yet the media may sometimes be a double-edged sword, employed as well or more effectively by opponents as by proponents. This is why supporters must take the initiative with the media, structuring news reports, presenting them in a timely and professional manner, and preparing arguments that effectively counter publicity created by the opposition. Based on our case studies, the most successful SBHCs are able to access trained public relations professionals for this purpose. Whomever controls the media controls the political debate and thus has a significant advantage in affecting public policy.

FUNDING FOR SBHCs

Long-term financial stability is the most important factor in the maintenance and delivery of comprehensive services by SBHCs. School-based health centers have been well supported in the past by private grants and some government funds. However, most often these funds were for start-up costs and not designed for long-term support. Grant monies have become less accessible for these programs after their first few years (Klein, Starnes, and Lotelchuck, 1990). As a result, SBHCs have had to become increasingly creative in patching together various sources of funds to meet their needs. Centers operate with a large variation in budgets, with a median annual operating budget in 1997-1998 of approximately $138,000. In a unique study of long-term financial viability of SBHCs in the western United States, Johnston (1998) found that almost 75 percent of the SBHC directors surveyed only had assurance of funds that would sustain their clinics for one to three years. Understandably, most of these administrators reported feeling uncertain and insecure, believing that attaining long-term viability for their center would be very difficult. Clearly assurance of reliable, ongoing financial support for these centers is a continuing and serious problem for SBHC sponsors (Dryfoos, 1994; Fothergill, 1998).

Johnston (1998) concluded that state legislative mandates and structures are necessary for centers to function. These mechanisms allow SBHCs to receive continuous annual government grant funds and to bill the state or federal government for services provided. Although states may have policies in place that allow health care providers to bill Medicaid for services, this form of reimbursement remains difficult for SBHCs because clinics are nontraditional forms of care and do not meet standard managed care criteria. States must approve legislation that facilitates the ability of SBHCs to seek traditional reimbursement and to contract directly with third-party payers and managed care organizations, and thus far only a slightly more than half the states have done so (Dryfoos, 1994; Johnston, 1998). As of the late 1990s an average of only 12 percent or less of SBHC budgets were derived from billing such sources (Fothergill, 1998; Schlitt et al., 2000).

Even with government support, financial structures for SBHCs will continue to be procured from multiple sources. A center's longevity is related closely to its relationship with institutions at the state and local levels. Thus, SBHC advocates "must become politically active. They must keep abreast of all the avenues available to them in order to create an environment that is supportive. This may mean having government representatives visit their centers . . . [and] personally lobbying for their cause" (Johnston, 1998:94).

Leadership and financial support at the state level have been the major catalysts behind the 1990s' boom in school-based health care. Just as states led the way in initiating health care and welfare reform measures that stalled at the federal level, they have moved to champion SBHCs as cost-effective and necessary providers of health care for youth (Making the Grade, 1995). State revenue allocations to school health centers increased dramatically in the 1990s to become the single largest contributor to clinic budgets. According to our 1998 national survey, state grants constitute an average of 36 percent of annual SBHC budgets, 2.5 times greater than the second largest single source, third-party reimbursements (14 percent). Even third-party reimbursements are most often from Medicaid, which is a largely state-funded health care program for needy, uninsured youth (and adults). State funds for youth health care were bolstered in the 1990s by new revenue streams, including increases in tobacco excise taxes in Arizona, Massachusetts, California, and Mississippi; monies from successful tobacco industry litigation in Florida; funds from video poker in Louisiana; and revenues from a sales tax on physical fitness membership fees in Florida (Making the Grade, 1995). The booming late 1990s economy, more than any other factor, filled most state coffers with budget surpluses, making it easier politically as well as financially to increase monies for school health care and other social needs.

As the focus of funding shifted to the state level, so did the political lobbying of SBHCs. By the mid-1990s, school health centers began to band together in statewide associations. State organizations numbered fourteen by 1999 and have proved helpful in communicating with legislators as well as bridging the worlds of managed care, state health departments, and school-based health (Making the Grade, 1999). In Louisiana, for example, where state monies for youth health care ranked among the lowest nationwide and where religious opposition to SBHCs was intense, a statewide assembly of school centers paid off. Organizing from the community level, the state association of SBHCs was critical in bringing the message of the vital role of school health centers for needy teenagers to the legislature and governor. According to the state director of adolescent and school health:

> They [the Louisiana Assembly on School-Based Health Care] have been really good at holding open houses and press conferences to bring legislators and community members into school-based health centers. And this has resulted in bringing in many opponents and turning them into friends. (Making the Grade, 1999:2)

State and local organizational and lobbying efforts in Louisiana achieved major successes, the most significant of which was a $2.65-million line item in the state budget in 1996 for SBHCs. This major increase in funding has been authorized annually since 1996, and shows that even in conservative southern states with active opposition, SBHC advocates can gain important state funding (Making the Grade, 1996).

CHARACTERISTICS OF SUCCESSFUL CLINICS

One way to investigate the components of successful SBHCs is to look at those clinics in our national survey that scored in the top tenth percentile on a composite index. This index combines the size of operating budgets, number of open hours weekly, number of services, size of recent service increases, rate of student usage, and number of summer hours. Although these may not be all the elements that would make for success, they include important indicators that can be combined to formulate a useful composite measure.

Examination of the twenty-one school health centers in the top tenth percentile reveals several characteristics that clearly set them apart from most clinics. First, all of the twenty-one SBHCs are located in large urban (80 percent) and suburban areas, not in rural settings where funding is more sparse. This reflects the prevailing trend to mainly address the problems of urban youth because disadvantaged youth are concentrated in urbanized metropolitan areas. Commensurate with this factor, there is a tremendous need for health care demonstrated in the neighborhoods in which these centers are found. Minority students, especially African Americans, are the poorest youth and have the highest rates of health risk behaviors. African Americans comprise an average 53 percent of the student population in these SBHC schools (as compared to 34 percent for other SBHC schools) (see Table 3.3). Clinic users are 79 percent nonwhite youth (contrasted with 60 percent rate in other clinics), and 76 percent of the students are eligible for the free or reduced lunch program (compared to 61 percent in other schools with clinics).

Another factor found common to these highly ranked centers is that they are found in relatively progressive states outside the deep South. With the sole exception of one clinic in New Orleans (LA), the other centers are located in states that are relatively affluent and supportive of school health centers. These states include California, Delaware, Florida, Illinois, Maryland, Michigan, New Jersey, New York, and Texas (Florida and Texas are considered border South states.) New York, which has by far more clinics than any other state in the country (158 as of 1998), claims five of these twenty-one successful clinics. Moreover, New York allocates more monies for SBHCs ($10 million in 1997-1998) than any other state, supporting 67 percent of all clinics in the state. In addition, seven of these ten states have state-

TABLE 3.3. General Characteristics of Most Successful SBHCs

	Most Successful (N = 21)	Average (N = 183)
Community Demographics		
Size of city (in thousands)	781	417
Percent African American	31	20
Percent Hispanic	15	13
Income	$14,240	$13,347
Percent poverty	22	19
Local percent Clinton vote, 1996	63	56
Percent college education	19	19
Percent conservative Protestants	15	23
School Characteristics		
Minority school board officials	12	4
School enrollment	2,038	1,134
Percent black enrollment	53	34
Percent Hispanic enrollment	27	19
Percent enrollment on free/reduced lunch	76	61
SBHC Characteristics		
Annual budget	$236,000	$133,680
Percent users of clinic	73	62
Percent non-Hispanic white users	21	40
Percent within state association of SBHCs	68	41

wide associations of SBHCs, which we have shown to be helpful in securing state funds and other forms of support.

These comprehensive clinics also receive high levels of support both within the inner circle of the schools and the outer circle of the larger community. Again, as we have previously demonstrated, local support is absolutely critical to the long-term success of SBHCs. As a clinic director from Michigan wrote in our national survey, the most important factor contributing to the maintenance and growth of her SBHC was "community support, first and foremost! The program director takes every opportunity to speak in and around the community to encourage support." Part of the process of building and sustaining such support is developing good public and media relations. Virtually all of these top centers reported several methods by which they communicated consistently with the news media and the vast majority reported favorable portrayals of their clinic activities by the media.

Having an active community advisory board was not essential, except for newly developing centers, but making sure that the board was inclusive of a great variety of community and school groups proved helpful. Furthermore, although a high level of support is necessary, these centers also experienced relatively little discernible opposition. Religious and political opposition in the United States tends to be concentrated in the South and in rural regions. These successful clinics were located in more progressive urban areas and states. Thus the percentage of conservative Protestants found in these urbanized areas is relatively low (15 percent) compared to other communities with school clinics (23 percent). Although some of these successful SBHCs had confronted opposition early on, especially resistance to reproductive health care services, clinic advocates proved adept at dealing with conflicts and resolving the issues. As a result, these centers have faced less opposition to reproductive health care than clinics elsewhere, but they also tend to avoid arousing resistance by not providing the most controversial of services.

Not only was political opposition less, but political advocacy was greater in these progressive urban sites. Large minority populations translated into significant black and Hispanic representation on local school boards. As Table 3.3 indicates, the average number of minority officials is three times greater in communities with successful SBHCs. Minority representatives are often zealous proponents of school health centers that serve largely black and Hispanic children, and their political power is a major factor of support.

In addition, these twenty-one highly rated SBHCs have obtained a high level of continuous, stable funding from both sponsoring organizations (such as local hospitals) and other sources. The average annual budget for these centers was $236,000 in 1998, more than $100,000 greater than the national average for other centers. Such financial support is absolutely vital for providing an extensive range of services to large numbers of needy students. It also has enabled these clinics to stay open full-time (forty-plus hours a week) not only during the school year but in the summer as well.

A final and very important ingredient for success is a committed, dedicated, and effective clinic director and staff. They are crucial to attracting students to clinic services as well as working with school personnel, families, and members of the community. In the words of a Chicago clinic director in a survey response:

> We recruit SBC staff who have a positive attitude about the work that is done with adolescents. The SBC staff have developed good relationships with students, their parents, the school principal, teachers, school counselors, and the school nurse. The staff have also established a sound relationship with our advisory board.

SBHCs THAT HAVE PROSPERED

Our case studies of SBHCs resulted in two sites that are considered relatively successful in terms of having many of the necessary components mentioned. The two school clinics are found in Portland (OR) and Albuquerque (NM). In each case, we trace briefly the establishment and development over time of the school health center, focusing on the elements that are important for success.

Portland (OR): A Model of Success

In 1984, Anne Cathey, a Multnomah County (which encompasses Portland) public health nurse, began to lay the groundwork for gaining public support for teen health clinics in Portland schools. She had recently attended a conference in St. Paul (MN) where she had observed a well-developed SBHC. Her proposal for Portland was based on the St. Paul model, especially its plan for community organization. At about the same time a member of the Robert Wood Johnson Foundation came to Portland to speak to community groups and to testify before the state legislature about the advantages of SBHCs. This action spurred a state legislator to propose a bill to fund several clinics throughout the state for high-risk youth. In the meantime Cathey and her colleagues convinced the Multnomah County Commission to fund a pilot SBHC for six months at a cost of $52,000. The first clinics were so successful that by 1988 the state was supporting six SBHCs, and Multnomah County had established three of its own clinics.

In Multnomah County, an urbanized metropolitan area with more than half a million residents in 1990, the superintendent of schools liked the idea of school health care for inner-city, low-income youth. There was also a deep concern by health and school officials regarding the problem of teen pregnancy. The health department opened its first center in Roosevelt High School in 1986 because the school had a large number of students with no health insurance and a high teen pregnancy rate. However, because of fear of opposition from the Catholic Church and Right-to-Life organizations to family planning services, the clinic opened without reproductive health care (Lear, 1996; Interview, Multnomah County public health official, December 5, 1991).

School-based health centers expanded throughout Oregon in the late 1980s. Growth was halted, however, when the state passed a property-tax limitation measure in 1990, and in 1992 state funding for SBHCs was reduced by 30 percent. Nevertheless, Multnomah County independently initiated and funded its own school health centers. Due in large part to the needs and resources of metropolitan Portland, the Multnomah County SBHCs had more staff and provided a wider range of services than most other health centers in the state (Brostrom and Hill, 1993).

The Parkrose High School Teen Health Clinic was opened in February 1990 as one of seven SBHCs sponsored by the Multnomah County Health Department. Its goal was "To provide comprehensive, accessible health services to a medically underserved population and to reduce the rate of teen pregnancy" (Stadell, 1989:1). The impetus for the clinic came from a county official who had heard of other such clinics elsewhere and was interested in establishing one at Parkrose. The demographic data, too, suggested a need for health services at the school. Thirty percent of the students were eligible for free or reduced lunches, a similar percentage were medically uninsured and had no other means of health care, and the teen pregnancy rate was one of the highest in the county (Zook, 1989).

The school's principal and its citizens advisory committee jointly requested the superintendent to solicit the school board's support to establish a clinic (Stadell, 1989). The Parkrose citizen advisory committee, composed of parents, also began to build support among other parents. Thus from its inception the primary representatives of the inner circle of support were engaged in clinic planning and advocacy. The school board, in turn, allowed ample time and developed a viable, well-managed process for community, student, and school staff input before voting on whether to grant the clinic contract to the county health department. Anne Cathey, the health professional and now teen clinic coordinator who brought the first SBHC model to the county, was invited to give testimony to the school board and at public hearings (Steineger, 1989). The school board requested that letters of information about the need for a health clinic be sent to all parents. Ultimately a community advisory board was established, as mandated by state law, and was composed of students, parents, school personnel, and a variety of community members. The board also included members of the opposition, a tactic that helped to reduce public criticisms. The advisory board was instrumental in reviewing clinic policy and activities, and encouraging community input and involvement (Interviews, clinic staff, December 5-6, 1991).

Another factor that supported development of the clinic at Parkrose was the news media. The Parkrose School District had an experienced, effective public relations office that worked in conjunction with its counterpart in the Health Department. According to a school board member, "Newspaper articles were objective, informative, and clear in terms of reporting events leading up to the opening of the SBHC" (Interview, December 5, 1991). Public relations and publicity generated by the health department were also helpful. For example, when the clinic opened, U.S. Senator Mark Hatfield, a moderate Republican, spoke at opening ceremonies, providing considerable publicity.

A significant amount of opposition surfaced at the public hearings, focusing primarily on reproductive health services. However, overall support for the clinic was well documented through carefully compiled local health statistics, a written survey of school staff and students, and a telephone survey of registered voters and parents in the district. The data indicated serious health needs of school youth including lack of access to regular medical care by one-third of students, high rates of drug and alcohol abuse, actual or fear of pregnancy by females, and suicidal ideation. Information from other clinic sites in the county demonstrated that they provided health care to adolescents who did not receive care elsewhere, and that teen pregnancy rates were lower in schools with clinics. Surveys showed that 81 percent of district staff and 77 percent of students favored the proposed clinic and that two citizens in the community favored the clinic for every one opposed. The school board voted four to one in favor of establishing a clinic, and several members mentioned that the survey results were a critical factor in their vote since board members had been exposed to a great deal of vocal opposition from constituents (Interviews, school board members, December 5-6, 1991).

The school board decision, however, was a compromise to expressed opposition as the board required parental permission for students to use the clinic and, more important, mandated no birth control distribution or abortion information. This decision was made despite the fact that the Parkrose survey showed that 59 percent of parents and 65 percent of community members favored reproductive health care. Furthermore, there was support at the state level where Oregon law stipulated that reproductive health services in SBHCs must include, at a minimum, family planning information and referral. As of 1992, state law also permitted centers to dispense contraceptives, but the Parkrose clinic declined to do so because of the fear of intensifying local opposition (Brostrom and Hill, 1993; Stadell, 1989; Interviews, school board members and officials, December 5-6, 1991).

Health services at the Parkrose clinic were somewhat limited at first, and attempts in the early 1990s to build a new high school and larger clinic failed in three successive bond issue votes. In response to the third rejection, the school board initiated a "visioning" process that involved extensive community participation in a series of meetings to discuss the needs of both youth and adults. The process helped to mobilize support for the ensuing plan. In 1995 a $35-million bond measure to construct a high school community center was approved. The promise of a school community center that featured a larger library, a performing arts center, a recreation center and pool, and an expanded health clinic persuaded voters that the new high school would now offer something for everyone (Stern, 1998; Interviews, school, community, and clinic officials, June 24-25, 1998).

The new, expanded neighborhood health center opened in 1997, furnishing more space, services, and health care for students, parents, and others in the community. The Parkrose SBHC had truly become a neighborhood health center, the first of its kind in the state. Its director, who has been overseer of the clinic since 1991, proved to be an effective advocate and coordinator of services. Trained as a nurse and adolescent medical specialist, she had gained valuable administrative experience as head of another SBHC previously. With increased funding from the county health department, the center added a full-time mental health therapist, a nurse practitioner, referrals for dental care, and became more active in preventive health care through classroom and clinic-based health education. There was also increased emphasis on reproductive care and family planning services, including HIV testing and condom distribution after school hours. The latter service was the result of a compromise with the school board, which had previously opposed any condom availability for students, but was in accordance with state law which mandated that county health departments provide family planning services to citizens, including youth aged fifteen and older without parental consent. The expanded family planning services were a response to the growth of a more diverse, poorer population in the east Portland suburbs surrounding Parkrose. By 1998 a quarter of the school population was minority (African American, Asian, and Hispanic) with relatively high rates of teen pregnancies, STDs including HIV, and 50 percent of students were eligible for federal lunch programs (Interviews, school and clinic personnel, June 24-26, 1998).

By 1998, the community health center at Parkrose enjoyed tremendous support from parents, many of whom used its services, and from students, teachers, and school administrators as well. The county health department continued its high level of commitment to providing health care for relatively poor youths and adults in the area, and funding for the clinic was at an all-time high of $288,000 per year (compared to a 1998 national annual average of $126,000 for an SBHC). By 2000 the school clinic had added more personnel, including a drug abuse specialist, and was truly a neighborhood access site, staying open two evenings a week (Interview, clinic director, July 10, 2000). The state of Oregon has maintained a supportive environment as well and is one of the top ten states in number of SBHCs with forty-one centers in 1998. Local health centers, moreover, have banded together in a statewide association (one of fourteen such organizations in the country) to communicate more effectively with state legislators and to share ideas with one another (Making the Grade, 1999). Although the community advisory board has dissipated, Parkrose maintains a schoolwide site council with representative parents and community members that consider various school issues including those involving the health center. Clearly the Parkrose clinic has been a model of success, building strong community and parental support, reducing opposition complaints, and providing a wide range of services that benefits the entire community.

Albuquerque (NM): University Outreach to a Poor Neighborhood

New Mexico was among the first states in the country to develop SBHCs due to its high rate of adolescent pregnancy and other poverty-related health problems. Statistics in the mid-1980s identified the state as having one of the highest teen birthrates and STD rates in the nation. Access to health services and to education about reproductive health care, particularly in many poverty-ridden rural areas in New Mexico, was extremely limited. These serious health issues raised concerns among health professionals and educators. In 1984 a dedicated nurse practitioner in Espanola, a small, poor community near Albuquerque, decided to expand the boundaries of her traditional role and established the state's first SBHC in the high school where she was employed. Family planning was included among the services offered by this clinic in an effort to address the high teen pregnancy rate. Responding to similar needs elsewhere and the documented success of the Espanola clinic, the state Maternal and Child Health Bureau began to dedicate resources to help form other SBHCs throughout the state in 1986 (Brostrom and Hill, 1993).

A large number of SBHCs soon developed in Albuquerque, the largest city in the state with more than 400,000 residents, 37 percent of whom are Hispanic. Utilizing a creative private-public partnership consisting of a three-way contract between the University of New Mexico (UNM) School of Medicine, the local public health department, and the school district, SBHCs were established in six schools. One of these clinics was set up at East San Jose Elementary School, located in an inner-city neighborhood that is more than 90 percent Hispanic. Most residents in the East San Jose community, one of the oldest neighborhoods in Albuquerque, were first-generation immigrants from Mexico with strong commitments to family and Catholicism. Half the students in the school had limited proficiency in English. The community was recognized as a "pocket of poverty," with

99 percent of its youth eligible for free or reduced school lunches and 65 percent living below the poverty line (University of New Mexico Health Sciences Center, 1998). Many of the problems facing residents, particularly children, of East San Jose were related to this pressing poverty. Drugs, alcohol, and gangs were prevalent, as was early sexual activity. There was a high incidence of teen pregnancy, mental illness, domestic violence, and a decaying community infrastructure. The vast majority of children in the community lacked any health care whatsoever, and many were undocumented immigrants who were ineligible for Medicaid. Thus, it was easy for health professionals and educators to justify establishing a clinic within a school serving this population.

Recognition of the profound health deficiencies of children in East San Jose resulted in the establishment of an SBHC in its elementary school in 1984. It was among the first such clinics in the state, and was designed as a feeder for the middle and high schools that would later enroll these youth. (These schools eventually procured SBHCs as well.) The clinic was initiated primarily by three individuals: the chief health officer for the school district, the school principal, and the chair of Family and Community Medicine at UNM. Each of these officials was extremely receptive to the concept of a clinic, and they soon gained the support of the school district superintendent and school board by promoting the goal of increasing access to health care for needy children. They also communicated with the state pediatric society and gained support from the medical community. The school nurse, who initially felt somewhat threatened due to her fear of displacement, ultimately became a supporter when she recognized that the clinic would provide additional crucial health services. The nurse was instrumental in getting parents involved in the planning process. When the nurse talked with parents about the health problems of their children, she would also mention the proposal for a clinic. Once informed, parents were supportive and, in turn, spread the word to others. Notices of public hearings were sent to the media as well.

A steering committee was formed composed of representatives from UNM Medical School, private sector organizations, and parents. This group planned and helped to develop the clinic. A community advisory board was established somewhat later, in 1987, but it was not very active at first. Gaining unanimous approval of the school board, the clinic was easily implemented with the assistance of the school principal and school staff. In general, SBHCs are perceived as less threatening at the elementary school level because few potentially controversial services are proposed. Moreover, parents in East San Jose were very involved in the planning process, and approximately 95 percent gave permission for their children to use the clinic. According to a school district health official, "At the elementary level, there is a different relationship between youth and their parents. Parents are more involved with and know more about their children than at older ages, and schools are more dependent on parents for information about their children" (Interview, April 20, 1992).

The role of UNM Medical School in the planning, advocacy, and implementation process for the clinic was absolutely critical. It provided funds, medical personnel, and other resources, and helped to mobilize physicians, nurses, and health professionals in the community. Indeed, the initial services at the clinic were provided by a physician, along with UNM medical residents (Interviews, April 30-May 1, 1992). School-based clinics generally are considered ideal sites for a number of departments within colleges of medicine to fulfill their service and teaching responsibilities (American Medical Association Council on Scientific Affairs, 1989).

In the early years, the SBHCs in Albuquerque, including the one in East San Jose, functioned relatively smoothly with little publicity or controversy. As is typical at the elementary level, the clinic provided basic and limited forms of health care including health screening and assessments, sports physicals, and acute medical care. Due to the city's large Catholic population, it was decided that most reproductive health care services would be unacceptable, and clinics at the middle and high schools neither dispensed nor prescribed contraceptives. However, providers in high school clinics did perform pregnancy testing and counseled students regarding, and referred students to outside physicians for, birth control. In 1987 Albuquerque's SBHCs came under broad attack by a coalition of fundamentalist religious organizations, antiabortion activists, and conservative political groups. The Catholic archbishop of Santa Fe also joined this opposition initiative that focused primarily on reproductive health care (Moore, 1987; Pacheco et al., 1991; Interviews, April 29-30, 1992).

The school board responded quickly and decisively, forming an ad hoc task force composed of a broad representation of parents, community members (including opponents), and school representatives to respond to complaints and mobilize community support on behalf of the clinics (Miller, 1987). The task force and the school board were ultimately successful in repudiating the right-wing attacks by rally- ing parents, teachers, students, and health care professionals, all of whom felt personally vested in the SBHCs. Previous attention to communications with parents had built a bridge of trust and solid sup- port for the clinics. In addition, many indigent families found that the clinics represented the major, if not sole, source of health care for their children. Indeed, the neighborhood Catholic Church remained neutral, recognizing the value of clinic services to their parishioners. School personnel and parents also realized that interventions by SBHC staff addressing family problems benefitted the entire commu- nity by helping to reduce truancy, drug use, and incidents of violence and vandalism.

Although much of the conflict did not affect the East San Jose Ele- mentary clinic directly, as it provided no reproductive health services, the community response bolstered its development (Pacheco et al., 1991; Interviews, April 29-30,1992; Rienzo and Button, 1993). As one local study of this political controversy concluded, "Through such strong school and community support, critics were perceived as outsiders pushing an unpopular, alien agenda. . . . As an outcome, the SBC movement came to symbolize local community control of its own affairs, and SBCs were strengthened and expanded" (Pacheco et al., 1991:94).

By the late 1990s the clinic at East San Jose had expanded services in general, including the addition of mental health care. The involve- ment of the UNM Medical School was again crucial in this effort. Additional physicians, a part-time social worker, and medical stu- dents in pediatrics from UNM provided clinical care. The longtime chair of the Department of Family Practice and Community Medicine continued to be a strong and dedicated advocate of school health clin- ics, and he supplied various resources from the School of Medicine at every opportunity. The Department of Psychiatry utilized East San Jose as a rotation site for its residents. The clinic gave greater empha- sis not only to primary health care but also to prevention of domestic violence and sexual harassment, and reached out through health classes that focused on nutrition, eating disorders, puberty, STDs, dental care, safety, and antiviolence. Primary funding continued to be provided by the UNM Hospital, but because of the large number of indigent users the clinic began to tap into Medicaid reimbursement as well.

In addition to UNM, community and school support have been the major factors that have contributed to the maintenance and growth of the clinic. The school board, the superintendent, the school principal, nurses, and health care providers from the community have all actively backed the SBHC. East San Jose's principal, a Hispanic, has particularly championed the clinic as a service provider to children with chronic, serious problems. As head of the school, his leadership and advocacy on behalf of the SBHC were essential. The activated community advisory board has represented various elements of the community including parents, the school board, teachers, health care agencies, physicians, nurses, and the school principal. It meets regularly (four times a year) and serves as an invaluable line of communication between the community and clinic staff. It also helps to identify the needs of students, keeps parents involved, develops new programs, and helps to secure additional resources. As an indication of the popularity of the clinic, the local United Way and city government have begun to offer support and funds (Interviews, May 3-5, 1999).

The coordinator for all Albuquerque SBHCs, a Hispanic female and former nurse who worked with children, has been a strong and effective advocate at both the local and state levels. She has worked well with both university officials and school and health professionals. The fact that there has been little conflict over reproductive health services, or any other issues, has also contributed to clinic success. In a small community such as East San Jose, citizens are informed about the clinic by word of mouth and through letters, consent forms, and flyers sent out from the clinic to parents. Virtually no media attention has focused on the East San Jose clinic because there is little controversy and the media is typically not interested in stories about "south valley poor kids" (Interview, clinic staff member, May 3, 1999). By 2000 the clinic had expanded its budget with a model Medicaid reimbursement program and additional funds from UNM Hospital.

Yet several significant barriers exist that prevent the clinic from fully providing the comprehensive services required to meet the needs of this community. The center attempts to alleviate almost insurmountable poverty-related problems (such as crime, drug and alcohol abuse, and domestic violence) on a very limited budget. There are a number of services, such as dental care and additional mental health services, that have been identified as priority needs but have not been incorporated to date. At the state level, officials have been mostly favorable toward school-based health services and there has been a steady expansion of existing programs. In 1992, the state allocated a small amount of money to initiate centers in thirteen rural communities. By 1998 SBHCs in New Mexico numbered forty, but state funding was relatively low (a total of $450,000) and clinic services were inadequate to meet student needs. Moreover, state dollars have targeted poor rural areas, not clinics in Albuquerque (Dryfoos, 1994; Making the Grade, 2000a). Cultural issues have affected the East San Jose clinic as well, with middle-class white health providers with limited training servicing poor Hispanic youth. The result sometimes assumes the form of language barriers and lack of mutual trust, or at the least misunderstandings related to medical recommendations and subsequent adherence to regimen (Interviews, clinic staff, May 3-4, 1999).

Nonetheless, the East San Jose clinic has clearly become a vital source of significant health and social care for some of the poorest children in the country. Furthermore, it has become an integral part of the school and community it serves, and is a model of university and community collaboration to solve pressing social ills.

Chapter 4

Sexuality Services
and the Political Opposition

State and local restrictions on the provision of reproductive health care and other sensitive services reflect the power of a vocal, conservative minority. These restrictions jeopardize the ability of SBHCs to meet the needs of adolescents.

Kate Fothergill, Director,
SBHC Support Center Advocates for Youth, 1998:39

A school health center "puts great pressure on young girls to become sexually active by offering contraceptives and abortion referrals while using a school campus setting to give promiscuity a false 'respectability.'"

Missionaries to the Unborn, 2000

Adolescents in the United States have had by far the highest fertility rates among teens in major Western, industrialized nations. According to the Alan Guttmacher Institute, a nonprofit organization specializing in reproductive health issues, 1 million teenage girls between ages fifteen and nineteen, 12 percent of that age group, become pregnant each year. More than half of the pregnancies result in births, most of which are unintended (Auerbach, 1996). In 1980, as SBHCs began to develop, the U.S. teen pregnancy rate of 96 per 1,000 females—compared to 45 per 1,000 in England; 43 per 1,000 in France; 35 per 1,000 in Sweden; and 14 per 1,000 in the Netherlands—was alarming. Even accounting for differences in the United States among racial/ethnic groups, e.g., African-American teenagers had significantly higher rates of pregnancy and births than did whites, did not explain the gap between the United States and other countries.

Likewise, teens in the United States and those in other countries had similar amounts of schooling and rates of sexual activity. Researchers concluded that the largely unintended pregnancies, like those among U.S. teens, were "*lower* in countries where there is *greater* availability of contraceptive services and of sex education" (italics in original) (Jones et al., 1985:60).

Teenage pregnancy has been considered a serious concern by public health officials in the United States because of the multiple and mostly negative ways it is associated with the future course of the lives of youth and their children. Commonly cited, the impact of pregnancy and early childbearing often includes the failure to complete high school and thus lowers earning potential for the parent, and medical problems, including abuse and neglect, for the children. In addition, escalating costs to taxpayers, an estimated $30 billion in 1991, serves to support the view that effective interventions are necessary (Zeanah et al., 1996).

In the early 1990s, the Centers for Disease Control and Prevention (CDC) began an initiative to measure the risk-taking behaviors of youth. This assessment, called the Youth Risk Behavior Surveillance System (YRBSS), produced data from surveys of youths in schools that could then be used to plan programs aimed at prevention of problems. The YRBSS conducted in 1999 revealed that 50 percent of all U.S. youth had experienced sexual intercourse by the twelfth year of school. Differences by racial/ethnic groups persisted: African-American teens were more likely to have engaged in intercourse (71.2 percent) than those of Hispanic background (54.1 percent) and white students (45.1 percent). However, the authors involved in this assessment, Kann and colleagues, carefully noted that "the association between race/ethnicity and certain risk behaviors is attenuated after controlling for socioeconomic status" (Kann et al., 2000:285). Although the overall rates of intercourse experience and teen pregnancy had decreased to some degree by the end of the 1990s (by 1996 the teen pregnancy rate had dropped by 15 percent from 1990) (National Campaign to Prevent Teen Pregnancy, 2001), CDC researchers concluded that "too many high school students nationwide continue to practice behaviors that place them at risk for serious health problems" including pregnancy and STDs including HIV (Kann et al., 2000:283). They strongly urged that these data be used to support public and school health prevention programs, especially for adolescents from low-income families.

Another strong impetus for provision of reproductive health care, including the dispensation of condoms, in SBHCs has been the increasing concern about HIV and other STDs among adolescents. By the mid-1990s, at least 25 percent of the15 million reported cases of sexually transmitted diseases annually in the United States occurred among youths. Indeed, every year three million teens, about 25 percent of sexually experienced youth, acquire an STD. Approximately 20 percent of all persons diagnosed each year with AIDS were likely infected during their teenage years. Although the CDC reported decreases between 1991 and 1997 in major risk behaviors associated with the transmission of HIV, it contends that many urban, particularly Hispanic and black, youth remain at high risk for the disease (Centers for Disease Control and Prevention, 1999). As a result, in 1997 the Institute of Medicine issued a recommendation that all school districts in the United States ensure that schools provide services including education, access to condoms, and accessible clinical services "such as school-based clinic services" to prevent STDs (Crosby and St. Lawrence, 2000:22).

SBHCS AND PREVENTION OF SEXUALLY RELATED HEALTH PROBLEMS

Most of the early discussion of school-based health centers emphasized their potential for reducing teenage pregnancy. In fact, one of the first SBHCs, developed in 1973 in St. Paul (MN), was created due to an obstetrician's concern about teenage pregnancy and was, at the beginning, solely devoted to providing reproductive health care services (Dryfoos, 1985). Subsequent to reports about this clinic's success in reducing teen fertility (from 79 births per 1,000 female students to 35 per 1,000 within three years), high rates of childbearing among students was repeatedly used as a rationale for initiating clinics across the country (Kirby et al., 1993; Santelli et al., 1992).

By 1985, family planning services were offered either on or near school premises in fourteen American cities, and the most highly publicized SBHCs were heralded as "pregnancy prevention programs" (Allensworth et al., 1997:409). Summarizing the admittedly little and mostly anecdotal data up to that point, Joy Dryfoos stated that SBHCs resulted in decreased fertility and dropout rates in areas with high rates of teenage pregnancy. Moreover, she contended that for areas with students demonstrating such risk behaviors "establishing [school] clinics may be one of the best ways to draw together the assistance that these children need to thrive, or even survive" (1985:75). In addition, a mid-1990s national survey of 1,200 students receiving reproductive health care indicated that those most likely to use SBHCs rather than going elsewhere for such services were minority youth living in rural areas (Crosby and St. Lawrence, 2000). Clearly, poor and minority students who have great needs but lack access to sexuality services are most dependent on school health centers.

In most of our case studies of school clinics, a chief motivation for considering the establishment of a SBHC was a high rate of teen pregnancies and STDs among students. In rural, predominantly black Quincy (FL), for example, local health officials noticed that a number of students were leaving Shanks High School to travel several miles outside of the city to visit the county health department. Their needs were primarily family planning, prenatal care, and treatment for STDs. Many students were not returning to school after their visits because of the distance and time involved as well as the lack of public transportation. In addition, school and health personnel were alarmed by the extremely high rates of infant mortality, teen pregnancy and birthrates, and school dropouts, and they realized the interconnection of these problems. Eighty percent of teen mothers dropped out of school because they had no one to take care of their child. In a county (Gadsden) in which almost 40 percent of youth lived in poverty with no regular health care, other student health needs were apparent as well. Providing easier access to health care, especially reproductive services, at no cost to the students was a major concern. As a result, local public officials recommended moving services provided by the health department into the high school in the form of a school health center (Interviews, March 25, April 8, 1992; Wooten, 1985).

In Jersey City (NJ), another predominantly minority city, health issues related to student poverty and high teen pregnancy rates were major factors in contributing to the initiation of a school-based clinic at Snyder High School. The advisory board's application for funding from the RWJ Foundation stated that many of the problems for which students sought help from school health officials were sexually related. Specifically, two of the most common health issues reported by Snyder students included pregnancy scares, actual pregnancies, and STDS. Thus the application listed "family planning, counseling, and screening" and "pregnancy counseling and, when needed, prenatal care" among the most needed services. Most students were receiving no treatment other than minimal care provided by the school nurse. In addition, the fact that 67 percent of Snyder's students failed to graduate suggested the need for a SBHC. Not surprisingly, the most controversial proposal by the clinic advisory board was the dispensation of contraceptives on site. For political reasons, the school board ruled against this proposal (Leir, 1986). However, once the clinic was established at Snyder, and an OB/GYN nurse practitioner was added to the staff, student visits for family planning and other sexuality services were among the most common (*Annual Progress Report,* 1991).

Highly anticipated, the first empirical study assessing births to teens in six schools with clinics was published in 1993 and concluded that birthrates were *not* significantly reduced (Kirby et al., 1993). However, a significant limitation of the SBHCs in this study was that none of them offered contraceptive dispensation on site. In that same year, the American Academy of Pediatrics claimed that "schools, by combining comprehensive health education and health services, can become sites for effective prevention of 'children having children'" (1993:307). Similarly, a summary of research in the area of pregnancy prevention found no evidence to support the contention by opponents that the presence of a SBHC *increases* the rate of sexual activity. The research demonstrated that clinics "had an impact on delaying the initiation of intercourse, upgrading the quality of contraceptive use, and lowering pregnancy rates, but only in programs that offer comprehensive family planning services" (Dryfoos, 1994:135).

The ability of SBHCs to offer contraceptive services, however, has been extremely controversial from the beginning and thus difficult to implement. The Center for Population Options, a nonprofit support program for school clinics, began collecting data regarding clinic services in 1985. In their 1989 results, the researchers noted that reproductive health care was a "highly sensitive issue" for SBHCs with only one in five (21 percent) dispensing birth control (Hyche-Williams and Waszak, 1990:7). A survey of 223 school health centers the following year revealed that only 15 percent dispensed birth control pills and 18 percent provided condoms on site. The vast majority of these SBHCs were located in high schools and middle schools where it was reported that "family planning services spark the most controversy" (Waszak and Neidell, 1991:14). By the late 1990s, little had changed in the ability of secondary school clinics to provide contraceptive services. In 1997, for example, fewer than 25 percent of SBHCs reported the provision of such services, and the survey report concluded that this continued to be a "key issue" for SBHCs (Fothergill, 1998:39).

Although providing birth control on site has been relatively rare, many SBHCs at the secondary level do address issues of reproductive health care in other ways. Our national survey found that 50 percent or more of the clinics at the high school or middle school levels offered services such as pregnancy testing, birth control counseling/referral, STD diagnosis and treatment, gynecological exams, and HIV testing. Fewer SBHCs provided the more controversial services of abortion counseling/referral (39 percent), birth control prescriptions (31 percent), prenatal care (21 percent), condom distribution (21 percent), and dispensation of other contraceptives (15 percent). As reported in the Advocates for Youth 1997 survey and the National Assembly's 1998-1999 census of clinics, 75 percent of secondary SBHCs are prohibited from dispensing some or all contraceptives either by state law or school district policies (Fothergill, 1998; Schlitt et al., 2000). Clearly these restrictions limit the ability of school health centers to meet some of the most crucial needs of adolescents.

Another sexuality-related need that is rarely met by SBHCs is sexual orientation counseling. A study of school clinics and sex education in Florida concluded that although issues regarding sexuality were given short shrift, "the silence surrounding the issue of homosexuality was deafening" (Emihovich and Herrington, 1997:160). Congruent with national studies (Button, Rienzo, and Wald, 1997), discussion of homosexuality in the classroom as part of sexuality education or any instructional curriculum occurred in few of the Florida schools studied. If the issue did arise, it was typically in the medical context of how the HIV virus is transmitted. Most clinic personnel were sensitive to the fact that more gay students were "coming out" and often facing a great deal of name-calling and harassment. They realized that gay students needed an infrastructure of support and the availability of counseling services. Yet the topic of homosexuality was so controversial in most communities that clinic directors feared that responding to the needs of gay youth might jeopardize their clinics.

According to our survey, only 38 percent of clinics provided counseling for sexual orientation issues. Our case studies confirmed the difficulty of implementing such services. In Albuquerque, for example, attempts to develop gay/straight alliances and to offer counseling services in high school SBHCs met with stiff opposition. Signs advertising the alliances and services were torn down, and the alliances failed in most schools for lack of support (Interview, May 4, 1999).

SOURCES OF OPPOSITION TO SBHCs

Over the past several decades, schools have become a major battleground over morality-based issues. Variously called culture wars (Hunter, 1991) or "morality politics" (Meier, 1994), the contested issues in this domain are distinctive because they are grounded in fundamental, moral concerns. In the case of school health centers, the primary moral conflicts have been waged over providing direct access to birth control, including condoms, and provision of information or counseling about abortion services. For many who are opposed to these sexuality services, the practices are viewed "as an affront to religious beliefs or a violation of fundamental moral code" (Sharp, 1999:3).

Because conflicts over reproductive health care derive from differences in basic values, the resulting political clashes are often extremely passionate and strident. Furthermore, the technical component of morality issues, such as reproductive services, is relatively low, thus allowing such issues to be presented in simple ways and to engage people who have no special knowledge of the topics. All of this suggests that many of the groups involved in this and other culture wars are not the conventional groups featured in local politics. Debates over sexuality services in schools mobilize additional forces. Chief among them are church leaders and religious organizations that have become prominently involved in this morality politics issue (Sharp, 1999; Tatalovich and Daynes, 1998).

Fundamentalist Protestants

The most significant opposition faced by proponents of SBHCs is from religious groups, and predominant among these is the conservative wing of Protestant churches such as Evangelical Protestants and Southern Baptists. School clinics, particularly the services related to sexuality, are perceived as a threat to the social values and cultural dominance of these religious groups. To religious fundamentalists, SBHCs are seen in the context of the growing erosion of social norms regarding sexuality and social restraint. In response many such conservatives have fallen back on the fundamentals of their faith and begun to mobilize politically against what they perceive as destructive social changes (Button, Rienzo, and Wald, 1997).

Protestant fundamentalists emphasize what they consider traditional moral values, including protection of the nuclear family, preventing abortion, and prohibiting premarital sex. In recent decades these religious groups have been organized politically—since the late 1970s, aroused initially by school textbook controversies, gay rights, and the Equal Rights Amendment for women. In each case, the religious right rallied to the defense of traditional social values. By the late 1980s many conservative Protestants focused their efforts at the grass roots, recognizing that the battles of deepest concern were at the local and state levels. Among their goals in local communities were challenging sex education and school-based clinics, and providing alternatives to abortion (Wald, 1997). Although many organizations were active in conservative Christian politics during this period, three stood out as the largest and best organized with state and local affiliates in most areas. These organizations were the Christian Coalition, Concerned Women of America, and Focus on the Family.

The most visible and active among Protestant fundamentalist groups has been the Christian Coalition. Founded in 1989, the Coalition boasted 1,700 local chapters in all fifty states by the mid-1990s. Its leader has been Marion (Pat) Robertson, a Baptist minister, television host, businessman, and former presidential candidate. Ralph Reed, a shrewd political strategist, served as executive director until the late 1990s. The Coalition molded an inclusive religious right, drawing support from all segments of the evangelical community. Politically, the Christian Coalition has had a broad conservative agenda and is active in every aspect of electoral politics, especially voter mobilization and in lobbying efforts (Moen, 1992; Wilcox, 1996).

Focus on the Family and its political arm, the Family Research Council (FRC), have also been active in the Christian Right. James Dobson heads the organization as well as a radio ministry broadcast daily over more than 1,500 stations. With an emphasis on pro-life, pro-family issues, FRC claimed some 100,000 local activists in twenty-six statewide affiliates by the mid-1990s. The organization specializes in gathering and disseminating political information, but it is also involved in voter mobilization and in attempting to shape legislation (Wilcox, 1996).

A longtime component of Protestant conservatism has been Concerned Women of America (CWA), often described as the "ladies' auxiliary" of the Christian Right. The organization was founded in 1979, developing at the grass roots through women's prayer and Bible groups. By 1994, CWA counted 1,200 local affiliates and a membership of several hundred thousand. Its issue agenda involves matters of special concern to women, including education, and it attempts to provide a counter to the liberal politics of the National Organization for Women (NOW) and other feminist groups. The CWA often works with the Family Research Council to disseminate information and voter guides (Moen, 1992; Wilcox, 1996).

Several other religious-based organizations have been active nationally, although they lack the grassroots presence of the previous groups. The Eagle Forum, headed by conservative political activist Phyllis Schlafly, is one of the oldest Christian Right organizations. The Forum was especially active in the 1970s fight against the Equal Rights Amendment, which eventually was defeated. More recently, the Eagle Forum has focused on education issues and opposing abortion through local lobbying activities. The National Right to Life Committee and hundreds of like-minded state and local groups emphasize their strong antiabortion position and often link that stance to religious belief. There is a good deal of overlapping of interests as most Protestant fundamentalists (as well as Catholics) are opposed to abortion, although they may not be formal members of any right-to-life organizations. Finally, there is the American Family Association (AFA) headed by Reverend Donald Wildmon. The AFA has helped to organize boycotts of television programs that contain extreme amounts of sex or violence or have an anti-Christian bias. More recently it has become involved in controversies over education issues, particularly school curricula and sex education (Wilcox, 1996).

In terms of party politics, these Protestant fundamentalists have proved active in the conservative Republican Party, particularly at the state and local levels. Indeed, by the late 1990s conservative Christians, having found that independent efforts had limited political effects, focused most of their political activities within the more mainstream Republican Party (Wald, 1997).

Battles over public education have been a major mobilizing force for all of these organizations associated with conservative Protestantism. The basic charge of religious fundamentalists is that the schools promote anti-Christian values and threaten the ability of parents to inculcate their children with their own values. One major source of the school problem, according to religious conservatives, is programs that promote "moral relativism." Sex education, reproductive services, and information provided by school health clinics are strongly indicted by Protestant fundamentalists who perceive such programs as dangerous to youth because they promote sex without fixed moral values, thus undermining religious beliefs about sexuality (Hunter, 1991). Although the conservative Protestant organizations that emerged to oppose SBHCs vary from one community to another, their basic rationale for attacking clinics is a common one.

All of the SBHCs that we studied in depth encountered opposition from religious conservative groups, but the most vociferous and effective effort by far was found in Virginia Beach (VA), the home base of Pat Robertson's Christian Coalition. Other opponents to the proposal for a school clinic in this city included the Virginia Society for Human Life, the Catholic Diocese of Richmond, Concerned Women of America, and the Eagle Forum, as well as some local evangelical church groups. In their arguments most groups cited their abhorrence toward the dispensing of contraceptives. As stated by one opponent in Virginia Beach, "Planned Parenthood will be setting up branches in schools" (Taped testimony, public hearing, April 29, 1986). Another claimed that a school nurse "told my daughter about oral sex without my permission, and told students where to get birth control information without parents' knowing. Schools shouldn't be doing this" (Taped testimony, public hearing, April 29, 1986). In addition, citizens attending a Virginia Beach public hearing to discuss plans for a SBHC expressed their fears related to the role of parents. "School-based clinics erode parental authority and involvement. They take children away from home and parents" and, in the words of another, "If the SBHC passes, our responsibility as parents will be eroded" (Taped testimony, public hearing, April 29, 1986). Another major issue was the belief that health care could be accessed elsewhere and thus the SBHC services would be a waste of tax revenue. All proponents of the school clinic concurred that political opposition was "very strong" and, in fact, "they killed it [the clinic]" (Interviews, March 9-11, 1992).

Since the mid-1980s religious conservatives in Virginia Beach have continued to limit the entire health program to one that offers less education and preventive care to students. A public health official stated that family life education (the school's sexuality education program) has become "very washed out due to Pat Robertson's influence." An opponent to sex education and SBHCs claimed, "We were able to change sex education and make it more conservative in tone and content. We now have one of the most conservative programs in the state" (Interviews, May 29, 1998).

In Portland (OR), Parkrose High School faced opposition from the statewide Oregon Citizens Alliance (OCA), a conservative political activist organization that tied in locally with fundamentalist—mostly Baptist—churches. School and public health officials also sensed the presence of the Eagle Forum and other right-to-life national organizations because the language from the local groups mirrored that found in publications by these national groups. Local conservatives appeared and testified at public meetings, making arguments reflecting a focus on their objection to sexuality services. Typical of their claims was that "SBHCs promote sexual activity" and "encourage kids to have an abortion" (Interviews, December 5-6, 1991). However, many of these opponents were known to come from outside the community. In response, the school board established ground rules that limited testimony to those citizens from the Parkrose district. Another tact that successfully documented the levels of support and opposition to the SBHC was the school board's sponsorship of a survey of citizens. This ultimately proved to be a key strategy because it showed that most of the Parkrose community was comprised of "silent supporters" and that the school's students and staff were solidly behind the clinic. As a result, the clinic was established despite the efforts of the opposition. Of note, however, were the compromises made to the opponents: the SBHC could not offer contraceptive services nor abortion referral, even though it was an arm of the local health department and legally obligated to make these services available to teenagers (Interviews, December 5-6, 1991).

Even the elementary level SBHC in Albuquerque felt the effects of Protestant fundamentalists. At its inception, fundamentalist churches "brought in bus loads from all over the district" to protest based on their conviction that clinics "sent girls for abortions and dispensed condoms" (Interview, April 30, 1992). This opposition was perceived to be backed by the Eagle Forum because that organization's literature was distributed, their arguments used, and their tactics followed. Also important, these opponents were identified as consisting mostly of outsiders who had no children in the schools where the SBHCs were implemented.

The Right to Life organization was particularly vocal and organized in Albuquerque. At a statewide pregnancy prevention meeting in 1991 their representatives stated that they opposed what they called "sex clinics" because they "encourage kids to use birth control and have abortions" (Interviews, April 30-May 1, 1992). Right to Life members were intentionally included on the Task Force, appointed by the school board, for planning Albuquerque's SBHCs and even filed a minority report to the school board. The effect of this opposition, however, was mixed. At the high school levels, the opposition resulted in the prohibition of birth control dispensation by the SBHCs. Proponents created the term school-based "health centers" instead of school-based clinics (the popular nomenclature at the time) because "clinic equals sex" (Interview, public health official, April 30, 1992). However, as in Portland, the opponents were revealed to be outsiders and this served to galvanize support in the community that became the basis of an "overwhelming vote of confidence for the school board to expand the health centers" (Interview, school official, April 30, 1992).

Black Evangelicals

Black communities are often divided to some degree in their views and support of SBHCs. A prevailing expectation is that African Americans are monolithic political liberals who strongly favor an activist government. As an identifiable minority subject to persistent discrimination, high poverty rates, and serious health and social problems, blacks have surpassed all other groups in their level of commitment to the Democratic Party. In this vein, African Americans have been strong supporters of public spending on social welfare and education programs (Wald, 1997). Black youth, as we have mentioned, have health problems that are more numerous and serious than other minorities and, in response to these needs, our national survey showed that black adolescents and children comprise approximately one-third of all youths served by school health centers. This proportion is significantly greater than for other minority groups.

On the other hand, many blacks are also committed to evangelical doctrine and an intense religiosity that has been a hallmark of white Protestant fundamentalism. Black evangelicals emphasize moral traditionalism, particularly in their views on a number of social issues. For example, black evangelicals oppose abortion and gay rights to about the same degree as white fundamentalists (Wald, 1997; Wilcox, 1996). To the extent that SBHCs offer counseling and/or referrals for abortion, and counseling related to sexual orientation, morally conservative African Americans tend to be less supportive of such clinics.

Nonetheless, the extent to which black evangelicals may actively oppose SBHCs depends on the nature of the local churches and ministers, and the particular public issues raised by school clinics. Black Protestantism contains "a strong prophetic component, a response to centuries of oppression." In this sense, Jesus is portrayed "as a force for liberation" and black theology becomes "a spur to social justice" (Wald, 1992:315). Thus for most black Americans, their religious commitment may well reinforce the liberal thrust of the black community, particularly on public issues of deep concern such as economic security, civil rights, and health care.

In Quincy, the black churches were a powerful political force and the primary form of organization and communication for African Americans. Early on the Ministerial Association, a local organization that included almost all black ministers, openly advocated the establishment of a health clinic at Shanks High School. Two black ministers, members of the Association, served on the planning committee and the first SBHC advisory board. The committee and board played key roles in building local support and in dealing effectively with the opposition. Jesse Jackson, the nationally prominent presidential candidate and minister, reinforced black community support when he visited the clinic in 1988 and urged parents and students to become advocates for the SBHC. For most black ministers, theology was preempted by the health care needs of poor black youth. As expressed by a black leader of the Ministerial Association and chair of the clinic advisory board, "I saw the impact on the lives of young people due to a lack of basic health services. Some youths hadn't ever seen a physician" (Interview, April 8, 1992). Although a small number of ministers maintained silence in the SBHC discussions due to their traditional views on sexuality, they did not actively oppose the Shanks clinic. All told, black ministers and many of their parishioners proved to be among the most avid supporters of the health center both in the short and long term (Interviews, April 8, 10, 1992).

In contrast to Quincy, the primarily black Ministerial Alliance in Jersey City was only one among several of the city's most powerful political organizations. Jersey City has a somewhat smaller proportion of African Americans than Quincy, and therefore relatively fewer black churches. Moreover, at the time the Snyder High School clinic was proposed, the Ministerial Alliance in Jersey City was in turmoil, divided internally over several religious and political issues. One of these contentious issues was the planned SBHC. Some black ministers favored increased health services for needy minority youth, yet others opposed the clinic based on their fears about birth control dispensation. As a result of this division, most black ministers and the Ministerial Alliance did not play an active role in the planning or maintenance of the Snyder health center. However, congruent with the political history of the Alliance, neither did they openly oppose the clinic. According to one African-American city official, "The Ministerial Alliance doesn't focus much on problems of the total community but on operational issues of the churches. Black ministers are sensitive to being seen by membership as supportive of controversial issues" (Interview, November 21, 1991).

Catholics

In some settings Roman Catholics have played an important role in the political conflicts over reproductive health care in schools. Catholicism is the largest Christian denomination in the United States, and sheer size alone suggests the potential influence of the church on this issue (Wald, 1997). Catholics have been drawn to the debate over

SBHC sexuality services because of their antiabortion and premarital sex positions. Some school clinics offer abortion information, counseling, or referral, but no SBHCs perform abortions on site. Nonetheless, some opponents have misappropriately labeled SBHCs as "abortion clinics" for their supposed role in encouraging abortion. Using this appeal, Evangelical Protestants have attempted to gain Catholic support in their crusade against school-based clinics.

Despite the clear stance of the Catholic Church, only a minority of Catholics are strictly antiabortion (or pro-life). Moreover, many Catholics are supportive of programs to aid the needy, including school health programs for disadvantaged youth. In spite of its reputation as a centralized church with a coherent theology, the role of Catholics on this issue varies from one community to the next. To some degree, this variation depends on the views of the local Catholic leadership (Wilcox, 1996).

In Albuquerque, where Catholicism is the predominant religion, secondary SBHCs came under attack initially because of the fear that they might provide reproductive health services. Fundamentalist Protestant groups and right-to-life organizations made up the primary opposition, as we have mentioned. Although the Catholic archbishop of Santa Fe spoke out against school health centers in general, there was relatively little mobilized Catholic opposition apparent in public hearings or at other times. This was partly due to the early decision by public officials that no contraceptives would be dispensed or prescribed at secondary school clinics. But the Catholic churches also remained neutral and did not actively oppose SBHCs because they recognized the potential value of the health services for poor Hispanic youth (Interviews, April 29-30, 1992; Pacheco et al., 1991).

Jersey City, too, experienced little political protest to clinic sexuality services from local Catholic churches. The state Catholic Conference registered its dissent to contraceptive services, but local Catholics played no political role in decisions that affected only predominantly black Snyder High School. As in the case of Albuquerque, the school board early on decided that no birth control would be provided at the clinic, so this issue was resolved almost immediately. Nonetheless, birth control dispensation surfaced again in the mid-1990s due to the increase in STDs, including HIV, among students. This time a Catholic priest who served on the school board led the opposition and the contraceptive proposal went down to defeat for a second time (Interviews, November 21, 1991 and May 19, 1999).

At Parkrose High School in Portland, the proposed health clinic attracted little organized resistance from Catholics. SBHCs established earlier in the Portland area, however, found opposition from the Catholic Conference severe enough to block the provision of certain reproductive health services. Lingering fear of more vocal Catholic political action, plus the outright opposition of fundamentalist Christian groups to family planning services, resulted in limitations on the Parkrose clinic. The local school board decided that no birth control dispensation or abortion information would be provided. Only in the late 1990s with increased rates of STDs and the dissipation of significant opposition was the Parkrose clinic finally able to make birth control available, although on a limited basis (Interviews, December 5-6, 1991; June 24-26, 1998).

Only in Quincy were Catholics a powerful political force that almost closed down the high school SBHC. The Catholic Conference mobilized its forces in nearby Tallahassee, the state capitol, and called for a town meeting in Quincy where Catholic representatives spoke against the already established clinic. Calling it an "abortion clinic," Catholics focused their opposition on the fear of abortion referral and birth control. Health professionals in Quincy attempted to assuage these concerns by emphasizing that abortion would not be discussed in the clinic, and that no services were provided without parental permission. Nonetheless, the Catholic Conference, with powerful constituencies across the state and well-trained lobbyists in the capitol, blocked state funding initially and then persuaded Catholic Governor Bob Martinez to physically move the Shanks High School health center off campus. This action, along with the governor's refusal to accept federal funds for a planned SBHC in a poverty-stricken Miami neighborhood, created national publicity (Seligmann, 1987). Local support was great enough to salvage the Shanks clinic, however, and with the election of a new governor the health center was returned to the high school. Unable to generate any significant opposition from parents or organizations in Quincy, the Catholic Conference ultimately withdrew from the political battle (Interviews, April 8, 10, 1992).

Parents

When parents publicly oppose SBHCs, the focus tends to be on loss of control and authority over their children. While parents' signed permission is required for SBHC services and is positively associated with successful programs (Allensworth et al., 1997), some parents object to allowing youth access to services, especially those related to sexuality, without direct parental involvement and notification. Of note, this opposition is often found among parents who do not have children enrolled in the schools with clinics. This source of opposition is effective, nonetheless, because it is often highly vocal and creates a public outcry that attracts media attention (Emihovich and Herrington, 1997; Rienzo and Button, 1993). Even though studies have documented parental support nationally for sexuality education and services in SBHCs, school officials are typically apprehensive about parental reactions to school involvement in programs that are sexuality related (Dryfoos and Santelli, 1992; Santelli et al., 1992).

To varying degrees, all SBHCs in our case study sites contended with vocal parental opposition at their inception. As a result, even though these opponents represented a minority of parents in their community (in Quincy, virtually all opponents were from outside the city and none had children in the clinic school), each of these SBHCs limited or completely abolished contraception and other sexually related services from their plans (Rienzo and Button, 1993). The results of our recent national survey reflect the persistence of some resistance by parents. As an SBHC director from Hawaii answered on our survey question regarding barriers to clinics: "Parents feel health issues are their responsibility. . . . They do not feel that people have the right to make their own choices."

In Portland, the Parkrose High School clinic finally gained permission to provide birth control in 1997 even though the clinic is an official arm of the local health department which, by state law, is required to provide such services to youth who need and request them. Even so, birth control is only accessible by students *after* school hours, which is a barrier because most students then have transportation problems. The clinic staff, who had been lobbying for this service for years because of the increasing needs evidenced by pregnancy and STD rates, agreed that this approval had to be gained quietly, for "if

publicly aired it would raise red flags among parents and others."
Staff want to offer similar services at the middle school level in response to pregnancies there as well, but the issue is "still seen as too
controversial" (Interview, public health official, June 30, 1998). Thus,
the level of sexuality-related services offered through SBHCs remains lower nationally than several other clinic services although the
need is great. Clearly when opponents to school-based health centers
show that they represent some parents, the ability of SBHCs to provide such services has been impaired (Rienzo and Button, 1993).
More recently, parental opposition has arisen to schools' provision of
mental health services as well.

A related complication for SBHCs is the legal regulations in most
states that allow minors to obtain diagnosis and treatment for certain
conditions, such as sexually transmitted diseases and mental health
conditions, without parental consent. Furthermore, minors are ac-
corded privacy for their medical records. Most SBHCs find a way to
work within these regulations to satisfy most of the concerns raised
by parents, students, school personnel, and insurance officials, but it
requires complex planning for carefully controlled and monitored
procedures (Allensworth et al., 1997).

CHARACTERISTICS OF CLINICS
OFFERING SEXUALITY SERVICES

What kinds of SBHCs are most successful in offering numerous
reproductive health services, often including dispensation of condoms and other forms of birth control? In contrast, what are the characteristics of school health centers that are prohibited from delivering
most sexuality services to youth and therefore offer few such services? The results of our national survey and our composite measure
of sexuality services enable us to identify the "top 10 percent" and the
"bottom 10 percent" of SBHCs. Since clinic reproductive health care
is offered primarily at the middle and high school levels, we focused
on SBHCs at these schools for this analysis and eliminated elementary school clinics from our respondent sample. This leaves us with a
sample of 175 SBHCs.

One of the most important characteristics of school health centers
that offer a vast array of sexuality services is their large urban concentration. Nineteen of the twenty-one most successful clinics are found

in urban settings such as Los Angeles, Chicago, Louisville, Baltimore, Portland, Houston, and Seattle. Seven clinics are located in New York City alone. From a public health perspective, there is an urgent need to provide reproductive health care to students in large cities due to their high risk of teen pregnancy and STDs. Indeed, a high proportion of poor (78 percent eligibility rates for free and reduced lunches) minority students, primarily African American (43 percent) and Hispanic (31 percent), attend these urban schools (see Table 4.1). As demonstrated previously, the highest youth rates of teen pregnancy and STDs are found among poor and minority youths. In addition to greater health care needs, urban areas are more culturally supportive of the idea of providing contraception to young people through school clinics. As Wilson (1995) has demonstrated, urbanism is associated with more tolerant attitudes about sexual behavior. Further, large cities tend to be more politically liberal and progressive than other communities, as suggested by the relatively high percentage of votes for President Clinton (67 percent) in the 1996 election. This compares to the 55 percent average Clinton vote in other communities with SBHCs (Table 4.1).

The age of SBHCs is also a factor that affects whether reproductive health services are offered, especially the dispensation of contraceptives on site. The older the clinic, the more likely it is to offer sexuality-related services, especially including family planning. Our survey results indicated that SBHCs providing the most birth control services (the top 10 percent) have been in existence nine years on average, while those centers offering the fewest such services (the lowest 10 percent) are almost 2.5 years younger. The National Assembly of School-Based Health Care (Schlitt et al., 2000) reported similar findings in their 1998-1999 census of SBHCs. Longevity thus reflects an evolution in programming whereby clinics tend to become more established and politically accepted within the school and community over time. They also become indispensable in terms of meeting the basic health care needs of poor youth. In this favorable climate, health centers are often able to introduce the more controversial services of family planning.

Socioeconomic status and level of education influence the provision of reproductive clinic care as well. Communities with higher per capita incomes (almost $6,000 greater than in the "least successful" clinic communities) can more easily afford an array of costly sexuality services (Table 4.1). Higher incomes translate into larger local tax bases, thus financing sizable SBHC budgets (more than $100,000 greater on average than annual budgets for clinics where few such services are provided). Higher levels of education, presented as the proportion of college graduates, suggest a citizenry that is more tolerant and understanding of the need for reproductive health care made readily available for youth. Nevertheless, multivariate analysis indicates that none of these socioeconomic and education variables rivals measures of political morality in explaining clinics' ability to provide family planning services (Wald, Button, and Rienzo, 2001).

TABLE 4.1. General Characteristics of Least and Most Successful SBHCs in Providing Sexuality Services

	Least Successful (N = 20)	Average (N = 134)	Most Successful (N = 21)
Community Demographics			
Size of city (in thousands)	306	317	1,001
Percent African American	19	21	23
Percent Hispanic	5	11	22
Income	$10,607	$12,893	$16,303
Percent poverty	24	19	19
Local percent Clinton vote, 1996	53	55	67
Percent college education	13	18	23
Percent conservative Protestants	41	23	10
School Characteristics			
Minority school board officials	6	4	9
School enrollment	1,034	1,184	1,418
Percent black enrollment	30	33	43
Percent Hispanic enrollment	12	19	31
Percent enrollment on free/reduced lunch	61	59	78
SBHC Characteristics			
Annual budget	$78,071	$133,468	$188,603
Percent nonwhite clinic users	49	58	84
Percent within state association of SBHCs	42	60	91

Without doubt, sexual health services are greatly influenced by morality politics. In addition to the effects of urbanism, the cultural values of the community exert a powerful impact. The availability of reproductive and contraceptive services is diminished significantly in communities with high concentrations of Evangelical Protestants. In communities where SBHCs offered the fewest sexuality services, conservative Protestants constituted 41 percent of all religious adherents. The proportion of moral traditionalists, therefore, is *four times greater* than in communities where school clinics offer the most comprehensive reproductive health care (Table 4.1). Controlling statistically for all other variables, the proportion of conservative Protestants was the single most important factor influencing the level of sexuality services (Wald, Button, and Rienzo, 2001).

Similarly, the South and Sunbelt regions, acknowledged to be the most culturally traditional regions of the country, are home to 90 percent of clinics offering the fewest sexuality services. SBHCs with a southern address also tend to be found in relatively conservative rural settings with the largest proportions of conservative Protestants of any region in the country. On the other hand, traditional moral values are noticeably absent in locations where one finds school clinics with the most reproductive health care. Such clinics are found mostly outside the southern region (86 percent) in progressive states such as California, Illinois, Maryland, New York, Massachusetts, Oregon, and Washington. These progressive settings are fertile ground as well for state political organizations of SBHCs. Thus health centers with the most sexuality services are commonly located in states that have statewide associations of SBHCs (91 percent). This compares to a 42 percent rate of state associations for school clinics that offer little reproductive health care (Table 4.1). Among other things, state organizations provide greater political power for SBHCs, often reducing state and local prohibitions on controversial sexuality-related services.

Clearly a culture war continues to be waged in many communities over the availability of sexuality services in school health centers. Not only do the data in Table 4.1 indicate a battle between moral traditionalists and moral progressives, but comments by SBHC directors to an open-ended question in our survey concerning "factors inhibiting the maintenance and growth" of school clinics reinforce this contention. Although lack of funding was mentioned most frequently in response to this question, the second most commonly cited factor was conservative opposition and citizens with false beliefs about reproductive services. A sample of the written comments by clinic directors in relation to this barrier is revealing:

- The widespread fear that SBHCs will corrupt youth with condoms.
- Right-wing political factions opposing SBHCs because of their supposed affiliation with family planning.
- Politically SBHCs are still controversial due to the continuing legacy of being thought of as "condom centers" or "sex clinics."
- Closed-minded individuals who do not recognize that teenagers engage in numerous high-risk behaviors, including sex.
- Ignorance . . . parents still want to believe sexual issues during adolescence are moral problems not developmental issues.
- Some are destructive with their religious agendas. They do not feel that people have the right to make their own choices in regards to health care.
- The clinic has a bad reputation for treating "pregnant girls and students with STDs."

POLITICAL TACTICS OF THE OPPOSITION

The opposition has been difficult to deal with because of their unconventional political tactics. In addition to the use of conventional forms of politics such as voting, lobbying public officials, and attending public meetings, opponents have employed a variety of other political mobilization techniques. Single-issue politics; the focus on issues that promote fear; and the use of religious symbols, public demonstrations, picketing, petitions, and highly charged pressure tactics have been common forms of opposition political activity. These unorthodox tactics appeal to groups new to the political process and therefore lacking in the resources, such as money and experience, necessary to make effective use of more conventional strategies. Moreover, mass actions, religious exhortations, and protests stir the passions of group members and attract media attention because they are unique and noticeable events.

These tactics and the nature of the opposition suggest a style of political conflict known as *identity politics*. This form of conflict is concerned with political issues that affect basic values and everyday life.

They are the values of primary identity such as race, gender, ethnicity, and especially religion, which for many defines their most fundamental values. When threats to these basic values occur, "they cut so deeply into the core of a society that their codification appears imperative, literally to 'save the world' as it has been known" (Mooney, 2001:4). For many conservative religious groups and some parents, school health centers represent a significant challenge to their traditional norms. As a result, these opposition activists turn to an array of political techniques, especially unconventional approaches, to thwart the efforts of clinic advocates.

The most common strategy employed by the opposition was to focus solely on issues of sexuality to arouse emotion and fear among parents and others who might potentially contest SBHC establishment. Almost every clinic opponent we interviewed at the five sites framed their objections in terms of sexuality issues, such as disseminating the belief that SBHCs encourage abortion, increase promiscuity, do not effectively decrease teen pregnancy, undermine parental authority related to reproductive health care, and freely dispense birth control (Rienzo and Button, 1993; Interviews, 1991-1992, 1998-1999). School health centers were commonly referred to as "sex clinics" or "abortion clinics". In Quincy, for example, the most frequently cited claims by clinic opponents were that a SBHC would "foster immorality," "increase teenage sex and pregnancy," "advise and perform abortions," and "hand out condoms" (Interviews, school and health officials, April 8, 1992).

Although all of these charges were misleading and most of them outright fabrications, opponents focused on the most controversial services provided by some school health centers, purposely ignoring the many other health services that had nothing to do with reproductive care. In addition to playing upon some of the gravest fears of adults regarding sexuality and youth, those battling SBHCs emphasized the loss of parental control to clinics, schools, and the state in terms of teaching youth about sex and reproductive issues. Potential loss of authority was also a significant concern of parents and other adults.

In addition, religious-based opponents often cloaked their charges in biblical language or religious predictions about the future, thereby further increasing the emotional tenor of the debate: Clinics are the "work of Satan," an indication that "God is being expelled from the school system," and in opposition to "God's word that 'sex outside of marriage is a sin.'" Others quoted passages from the Bible to support their claims and read prayers at public meetings expressing hope that SBHCs would not be established (Rienzo and Button, 1993; Interviews, 1991-92). This strategy not only helped to mobilize more traditional parents and citizens but also intimidated some public officials. In the words of a Virginia Beach city council member, "It's awfully hard to be against God" (Interview, March 11, 1992).

Manipulation of public meetings where SBHCs were discussed was another political strategy employed by opponents. "Packing" such meetings with large, sometimes unprecedented numbers of citizens, often bused to the meetings in church-owned vehicles, was used to demonstrate the organization, size, and strong feelings of those opposed. Many parents brought their children with them and some youth were urged to speak publicly as well. Often citizen and prominent leaders from outside the school district and even outside the region were mobilized to attend public meetings to increase numbers and provide testimony.

Thus attendance and presentations at public hearings were carefully orchestrated by the opposition. In Portland, for example, the presence of the opposition at public meetings was like a "staged media event" (Interview, public official, December 5, 1991). Using a telephone tree staffed by retirees to contact and mobilize people, those who objected to SBHCs filled the meetings. They distributed pamphlets that presented their arguments both at the meetings and in school neighborhoods. Designated spokespersons included parents and local citizens, many with planned presentations, and "experts" imported from regional or national conservative organizations. These external organizations also provided literature and money to support SBHC adversaries.

Protests, picketing, and petitions were common tactics employed by opponents as well. Organized groups attempting to block SBHCs often displayed signs at and picketed public hearings, school board meetings, and schools designated for a clinic. The press was contacted and television stations were notified in advance to guarantee media coverage. Petitions were commonly circulated among opponents and then presented to school board members and other public officials. Numerous letters to the editor were printed in local newspapers, and large amounts of mail were sent to city and school administrators. "I received thousands of letters and postcards . . . stacks of mail . . . and many phone calls too . . . more than one contact from each opponent, I'm sure," claimed a Virginia Beach school board member shortly after the SBHC controversy there (Interview, March 9, 1992).

The opposition also attempted to intimidate public officials by threatening to defeat future school bond issues, organize school board recall elections, create state legislation to cut or eliminate clinic funding, and file lawsuits (Rienzo and Button, 1993). Few of these threats materialized, but they did have an impact on many officials. "I felt tremendous pressure from my church [Catholic] and even my friends and relatives on this issue," stated an Albuquerque school board member (Interview, April 30, 1992). In Quincy, after weeks of political pressure and several threatening phone calls, a longtime public health officer claimed, "I feared I was in danger of losing my job" (Interview, April 8, 1992).

Although political conflict over reproductive health care was most intense during the establishment and initial years of SBHCs, opposition to sexuality services and programs continued throughout the 1990s. Due to significant political resistance, especially from the religious right, the decision was made early on to prohibit the on-site provision of birth control and various other services at most clinics. Intimidated by opponents and unaware of how to respond effectively to their unusual strategies, many advocates retreated from the most controversial issues of reproductive health. When such issues did arise due to the increasing needs of poor and minority youth (particularly increased rates of HIV/AIDS) or for some other reason, sexuality services were quickly contested by the same conservative forces and in the same political manner as in previous times.

At the Parkrose clinic in Portland, greater community support and politically experienced advocates enabled the health center to reach an agreement with the county commission and school board in the late 1990s to dispense birth control. Nonetheless, some parents and fundamentalist church groups surfaced to oppose the provision of birth control and forced the SBHC to a compromise agreement which made such services available only after school hours (Interviews, June 25, 26, and 30, 1998). In Jersey City, Albuquerque, and Virginia Beach opponents remained sufficiently active to keep the most controversial sexuality-related services and programs off the local political agenda during the decade.

By the mid-1990s, conservative—especially religious—forces increasingly shifted their efforts to the state level where greater funding and reproductive health programs for SBHCs were being debated. In Virginia the Christian Coalition and the local branch of Focus on the Family were successful in lobbying state legislators to mandate a more conservative sex education curriculum. Due to pressure from the Christian Coalition, Louisiana's legislation which authorizes SBHCs prohibits dispensing contraceptives or counseling for abortions on site. In the late 1990s the Coalition pushed state legislation to stop clinic referrals for and counseling about contraceptives, but well-organized advocates were able to defeat this initiative (E-mail communication, Louisiana SBHC official, June 23, 1997). "We are constantly battling the Christian Coalition," claimed a Baton Rouge (LA) school health center director. "They have a huge influence on politicians at the state level" (Telephone interview, January 5, 1999).

The use of unconventional political tactics has often been effective because clinic advocates were not accustomed nor prepared to respond to such unusual strategies. As a result, proponents often found themselves on the political defensive, attempting to answer charges and to fend off the attacks of the opponents. Those opposed to SHBCs have been in control of the political contest, at least until advocates began to learn how to play the new game of politics. Thus morality issues and identity politics introduced new ways of waging political war, providing many advantages to opponents.

STRATEGIES OF ADVOCATES

As we have seen, the opponents of reproductive services in school health centers, especially religious conservatives, perceive the battle over SBHCs as one between right and wrong. In the quest to preserve their traditional values, opponents have resorted to a variety of conventional and unconventional political tactics. The unpredictable nature of such tactics, plus the employment of protest and other nonconventional strategies, has often found advocates surprised and unprepared for political conflict. This was especially the case during the early period of school health clinic development before health and education professionals learned from their experiences and developed strategies to contest these tactics.

Because morality politics involves conflicts among those with absolute positions, compromise on policies is highly unlikely. Thus advocates of reproductive health care have come to realize that even the best of arguments and information concerning the advantages of school clinics will not sway the entrenched opposition. Persuasive tactics must therefore focus on other community groups and individual leaders who are potentially interested in and open to new approaches to sexuality services for youth. These interests are the "undecided majority" that will often be decisive in the battle of absolutists. Involving parents, students, educators, health and social service professionals, minority groups, politicians, and others in the conflict, and convincing them that school health centers are important, useful programs, are essential steps if proponents want to prevail. This realization is crucial because advocates and opponents in morality politics often spend much of their efforts focusing on each other, or "fighting the enemy," rather than involving the silent, yet significant, majority.

Advocates have employed and found effective several strategies in gaining support from undecided groups and citizens. Early on, it is extremely important to gather extensive, reliable data on student health and reproductive care needs. This is best accomplished through a needs assessment survey of students and/or parents (parents are preferable when young children are the target population). It may be augmented with state and/or national data, but it is essential to have the health problems and needs of local youth documented. In all of our case study communities with a SBHC, various assessments of youth health care needs were conducted. Most important, the results were widely publicized throughout the community as a way to convince the uninformed, noninvolved public of the need for school health centers. According to a leading health professional in Albuquerque, "The needs assessment should be broad in scope, exploring a variety of health issues so that the opposition cannot focus on just one (like sexuality issues)" (Interview, April 30, 1992). Added another health official, "We used the survey results to document the need for health centers in schools where most children live in poor families . . . where a SBHC is almost a necessity . . . and where kids get no other health care" (Interview, April 20, 1992).

Publicizing the health care—including reproductive care—needs of youth, and the reasons that a school-based clinic is an ideal approach for meeting these needs, is another important strategy. Educating parents and the broader community about youth health issues and the record of SBHCs in reducing the identified problems is vital. It is also important to publicize the fact that parents have ultimate control over their childrens' use of the clinic because formal parental permission is necessary. Public forums, letters to parents, presentations to civic and other community groups, and proactive use of the media are proven methods for informing the public. Media coverage, in particular, is significant. A proactive approach enables clinic advocates to avoid emphasis on "sex issues," which some media representatives wish to exploit, and to focus on the many ways that SBHCs are "good for kids" and that "health is inexorably linked to learning" (Interview, public health official, Portland, June 30, 1998).

Another strategy employed by advocates is to introduce SBHCs first at the elementary school level where sexuality-related services are not an issue. As children graduate to higher grade levels and the SBHC proves its value, their parents will often come to expect, and actively support, the continuation of school health services. Ultimately youth and parents become stakeholders defending their "entitlement" at the high school level where the deficiency of reproductive services becomes most clear. Having built a constituency for such services and a high degree of trust and confidence within the community generally, SBHCs find it considerably easier to offer controversial sexuality services (Interview, Albuquerque, May 4, 1999; Marone, Kilbreth, and Langwell, 2001).

A similar incremental approach is to initially develop SBHCs at higher grade levels but with no reproductive health care. The emphasis would be on the delivery of primary, and necessary, health services. This modest, scaled-down plan normally attracts little or no opposition or negative publicity. Once the school health centers are well-established and have gained a reservoir of support, they can proceed to introduce the more controversial but essential reproductive care services. This may be done "quietly and without fanfare," beginning with the least contested services (Interview, SBHC director, rural New York community, February 15, 1999). This "stealth" approach enables clinic personnel to test the political waters in an incremental fashion to see what the nature and strengths of the local opposition are before proceeding with a full range of reproductive health care services.

Finally, mobilizing "experts" on youth and health care, such as well-known medical doctors, nurses, and hospital personnel, to testify publicly about the positive aspects of SBHCs is a sound approach. The opposition often promulgates erroneous information about school health centers to influence and frighten citizens who have little knowledge of such centers. It is crucial to counter the false claims of opponents, as well as to be proactive in general, by utilizing expert testimony based on personal experience and knowledge of published studies of SBHCs. In addition to local experts, who are easiest to enlist and typically have a great deal of influence and credibility in the community, state and even national authorities are often beneficial. Advocates in Quincy, for example, brought in a representative of the RWJ Foundation, a man with considerable experience in school clinic development, who gave advice and public talks that proved "invaluable" (Interview, public health official, April 8, 1992). Nationally known presidential candidate Jesse Jackson and Florida Governor Lawton Chiles also visited and endorsed the Shanks clinic. These actions by national leaders gained a great deal of media coverage and local attention, and were instrumental in informing and influencing local citizens who had not yet taken a position on the health center.

All of these strategies presume solid support for SBHCs from the inner circle of school personnel and administrators, as well as the school board and superintendent. It is virtually impossible to convince various community groups and individuals of the need for school health centers without the strong endorsement of key school officials and personnel.

As the focus of clinic funding and regulations shifts to the regional and state levels, so does the opposition (Center for Health and Heath Care in Schools, 2000). This requires that SBHCs with sexuality services develop regional or statewide associations to publicize and build support for clinics across communities and at the state level. Enrolling appropriate state officials from the departments of health and of education, and supportive state legislators, is an important part of building a necessary statewide coalition of advocates. At the state as well as local level, it is crucial to "out organize" the opposition to gain broader support and win the moral battle.

RACE AND POLITICS MATTER

The staunch political resistance to SBHC reproductive health care services is not easy to overcome. The demonstration of severe needs of youth is necessary but not sufficient. Thus sexuality services are most likely to be offered in communities with large proportions of poor minority students who are perceived to be at high risk of teen pregnancy and STDs. Yet communities where SBHCs provide relatively little reproductive health care also have grave youth needs as indicated by the higher-than-average community poverty rate (24 percent) and percentage of students enrolled in the free/reduced lunch program (61 percent) (Table 4.1). This suggests that health care needs alone do not determine whether a school clinic provides ample sexuality services, and further analysis of our data confirms this (Wald, Button, and Rienzo, 2001).

What matters is the race of the students. Minority students, particularly those who are black, are most likely to receive controversial sexuality services. Indeed, nonwhites make up 84 percent of clinic users in those SBHCs offering the most reproductive health care, whereas white students are the majority (51 percent) in clinics providing few such services (Table 4.1). Those in political power, most often white officials even in minority-dominated school districts, believe that minority students are at high risk sexually. Yet they also know that providing reproductive health care, including dispensation of condoms and birth control, to black youth engenders much less political opposition than when those students in need are white. Clearly this is a redistributive policy that is rare in American politics; that is, providing *greater* resources to predominantly black and Latino schools than to schools filled with lower-income white students. Certainly the demographics of minority schools, large cities with relatively few religious conservatives, facilitate this redistributive policy. However, race is also an important consideration. Conservative opponents to sexuality services seem willing to compromise their religious concerns when minority students are considered. What matters most is a race issue consisting of fears that black (and Latinos to a lesser extent) teens will reproduce at a high rate, thus increasing the proportion of African Americans in society, and that black teen mothers will become welfare recipients, thus increasing costs for taxpayers.

In Jersey City, for example, there was generally strong opposition to the distribution of birth control through SBHCs. According to a city official, however, Snyder High School, "because it was African-American, didn't have much opposition." This official further explained, "It was important that a clinic was proposed for Snyder High School first, with its predominantly black population. The SBHC would not have been accepted in another school that was not black" (Interview, November 21, 1991). Public officials in Quincy, too, claimed that the lack of local opposition to a SBHC with reproductive health care was due to the commonly held perception by whites that teen pregnancy was a black issue that needed attention. Most white students were enrolled in private schools since school desegregation. Therefore the clinic at Shanks High School, whose enrollment was 90 percent African American, was not an issue for white adults who normally would have opposed such services for white youth (Interviews, April 10, 1992).

Race influences the provision of sexuality-related services for minority students in another way as well. Research suggests that political representation of blacks and Hispanics on school boards often has an impact on school policies that favorably affect minority students (Meier, Stewart, and England, 1989; Meier and Stewart, 1991). Our data support this contention as well with minority school board members in districts where SBHCs offered numerous sexuality services averaging almost twice the number of those in districts where clinics provided few such services (Table 4.1). Black and Latino school board officials not only advocate directly for greater services for minority students but also push to appoint or hire more minority school administrators and teachers who in turn become advocates for black and Hispanic youth.

Quincy proved to be a fine illustration of the key role of minority officials in SBHC politics. When the Shanks High School clinic was in its planning stages, African Americans served as the elected school superintendent and as two of the five school board members, including the board's chair. Both the superintendent and school board chair were strong, outspoken advocates of the health center, including the provision of reproductive health care. The superintendent worked to gain the support of the county commission, which was asked to fund the clinic through its public health department. The black superintendent and school board officials also helped to build a community network of support. When controversy arose over sexuality-related services that would be provided by the clinic, the school board chair "took the heat" for this and publicly defended the importance of such services (Interviews, school and health officials, April 8 and 10, 1992).

In Jersey City, an African-American school board member (one of four minorities on the six-member board) was crucial to the development of the Snyder High School clinic and the variety of reproductive health care services provided there. The school board official, aware of the needs of black and Latino youth, helped to develop the initial proposal for the health center. She also helped to involve black parents and students in the process and made sure several were appointed to the clinic's advisory board. In addition, the black school board member elicited the support of the local NAACP and the media, inviting a "friendly" newspaper reporter to public meetings where the SBHC was discussed. Similarly, the black school board superintendent and black Snyder High School principal were instrumental in explaining the importance of the clinic to the public, and in getting the African-American churches and PTA behind the health center. The active support of these black officials had "a real calming effect and defused or deflected potential opposition" (Interview, November 22, 1991).

Chapter 5

The Future of SBHCs
As a School Reform:
Issues and Recommendations

These developments [the tremendous growth of SBHCs in the 1990s] make the transition of school-based health centers from the margins to the mainstream of the American health care system.

Julia Graham Lear, 2001

School-based health centers have grown dramatically over the past decade, from approximately 200 in 1990 to almost 1,400 in 2000. SBHCs are now found in forty-five states plus the District of Columbia. Notably, recent census data show extensive growth has occurred in traditionally conservative states, such as those in the Sunbelt (Arizona, Mississippi, West Virginia) and in the Midwest (Ohio, Wisconsin, Missouri). Similarly, most recently established SBHCs are in suburban and rural communities, where many whites previously had perceived little need for school health centers. Finally, a number of new school health centers have been placed in elementary and middle schools. This growth and expansion into new domains suggests that SBHCs have survived the demonstration phase and have become a valued health service delivery model for many children and adolescents (Schlitt et al., 2000).

Clearly, SBHCs have successfully garnered substantial support in communities throughout the United States. At the same time opposition to school clinics seems to have lessened. The most recent census of SBHCs (Center for Health and Health Care in Schools, 2001) reported that those in thirty-six states had been asked for information on how to start, operate, or fund clinics, while those clinics in only thirteen indicated that they had been contacted by persons who opposed SBHCs. In addition, state-level support has increased significantly as well. State funding for SBHCs rose from $17 million in 1992 to $61.9 million in the 1999-2000 school year (Lear, Eichner, and Koppelman, 1999; Center for Health and Health Care in Schools, 2001). Nonetheless school health centers continue to face several important issues that have limited their effectiveness.

FINANCIAL SUPPORT

Despite the significant increase in funding and political support for SBHCs in the 1990s, lack of sufficient finances is still the foremost issue afflicting clinics. Recent surveys have indicated that billing third-party payers for school health center services is increasingly common. Nonetheless, many students are uninsured or underinsured, and Medicaid and other forms of third-party reimbursement remain "an elusive and complicated means of financial support" (Schlitt et al., 2000:191). Furthermore, local tax bases in poor neighborhoods typically served by SBHCs are too low to adequately fund school clinics.

Increasingly the support, financial and otherwise, for school-based health care is coming from state governments. In fact, Lear, Eichner, and Koppelman (1999) reported that more than half of the states with SBHCs have developed a governmental unit explicitly charged with supporting their centers, and that the vast majority of those have formulated official standards for operating SBHCs. Only eight states with centers do *not* provide specific funding mechanisms to support their SBHCs, and all the states with the largest numbers of centers provide such earmarked financial assistance. State funding for school clinics primarily comes from state general funds and state allocations from federal Maternal and Child Health block grant dollars (Making the Grade, 2001).

Nonetheless, as the demand for health services, including school health centers, for uninsured youth has grown, many states have been overwhelmed by requests for funds. In Arizona recently, the state Department of Health Services received $18 million in grant solicitations for SBHCs. The state, however, had set aside only $6 million of tobacco-tax revenues for school clinics. As a result of the shortage in state funds, a number of Arizona's 116 clinics—the primary source of health care for many of the state's 342,000 uninsured youth—have been forced to cut back services or close (Bland, 2001). In New York City, officials may also have to shut down more than two dozen school-based and neighborhood health clinics due to huge deficits and inadequate state support (Sengupta, 2001).

In addition to making increased demands for limited funds, SBHCs have faced another major hurdle in gaining more state dollars. The 1990s saw a dramatic shift in partisan politics at both the federal and state levels. The Republican Party captured both houses of Congress and majority control of legislatures in eleven new states in 1994. By 2000 the GOP held a majority in more state legislatures than the Democrats for the first time since the 1950s (National Conference of State Legislatures, 2001). Republicans also won fifteen new governors' offices between 1993 and 1996, and by 2000 controlled twenty-nine governorships. Most Democrats had embraced school health centers, but more conservative Republican politicians have not been willing to make the same kind of commitments. In North Carolina the new Republican-majority legislature forbid any of the State Children's Health Insurance Program (SCHIP) funds from going to SBHCs. Louisiana's Republican governor, backed by the Christian Coalition, attempted to abolish (without success) school health centers (Marone, Kilbreth, and Langwell, 2001).

Health care providers and educators, however, are learning how to successfully play interest group politics at the state level. As the devolution of power from Washington shifted increased federal health care funds and responsibility to the states, SBHC advocates have begun to lobby state legislators. Statewide associations of school health centers have been organized, and groups of parents, students, teachers, and health care providers now travel to the state capitol to make their case. In addition, state health administrators and even governors are increasingly joining local activists as SBHC advocates. We found bureaucratic activists in state health departments in New Jersey and New Mexico who were lobbying state legislators and helping to guide local school and health officials through the political process at the state level (Interviews, state officials, New Jersey, June 21, 1999; New Mexico, May 5, 1999). In Delaware, Governor Tom Carper helped to establish a SBHC in nearly every high school, and New York's Republican Governor George Pataki strongly supported the state's annual allocation of $18 million to some 159 centers (Making the Grade, 2001).

Advocates have learned how to appeal to state legislators with arguments that SBHCs provide ideal constituent services. Simply put, school health centers combine education and health care; meet primary health needs of the poorest youth yet are increasingly valued by middle-class suburban parents; are cost effective and a relatively inexpensive budget item; and are locally delivered services that avoid the bureaucratic red tape that engulfs many other health services. This message has a broad appeal to legislators that cuts across partisan boundaries. By the late 1990s increasing numbers of Republican politicians were adding their support to SBHCs (Marone, Kilbreth, and Langwell, 2001).

Recent developments have made state coffers the ideal place to look for enhanced funding for SBHCs. With the enactment of the State Children's Health Insurance Program (SCHIP) in 1997, the federal government made available $40 billion over ten years for states to provide health care coverage for millions of uninsured children. Although initial state activity to utilize SCHIP funds was slow, by 2000 state use of this large federal allocation had accelerated. Important for school health centers, SCHIP monies can be used to help youth enroll in any government-funded or private health program (Meyer and Silow-Carroll, 2000). In middle schools and high schools, where many low-income children have been either too old to qualify for Medicaid or not quite poor enough, SBHCs report that almost half of the students they care for are uninsured and eligible for SCHIP funds (Koppelman and Lear, 1998).

An even greater financial windfall for states is the 1998 tobacco industry settlement that calls for $246 billion in payments to states over the next twenty-five years. With initial payments totaling $13 billion in the first five years, along with $4.5 billion in annual allocations that began in 2000, the states are flush with new funds that have few strings attached. With the obvious connection between smoking and health care, some thirty-eight states allocated $4 billion for health programs and research in the fiscal year 2000-2001. This amount was almost half of the $8.2 billion total outlay for this period, and by far the largest share of the settlement money (Greenblatt, 2000). Lobbying for this tobacco money is intense, but the focus on health care provides an advantage to SBHC advocates. As of 2000, several states, including Florida, Illinois, Louisiana, Massachusetts, and Mississippi, had devoted a portion of initial tobacco funds to school health centers (Making the Grade, 2001).

Another source of funding for SBHCs in poorer school districts has been the impact of state-level school finance litigation. Given the great disparities in school funding found in many states in the 1980s and 1990s, litigators have pursued claims for more equality in school finance at the state court level. Winning in twenty of thirty-six states (some decisions are still pending), legal activists have forced state legislatures to enact reforms that provide greater resources to poor school districts. In states such as Texas, Kentucky, New Jersey, Connecticut, Tennessee, and others, court-initiated school financing decisions resulted in greater equalization in funding (Reed, 1998). Other states such as Michigan and Nebraska moved independently to reform funding distributions.

In all cases of school finance reform the increased attention given to poor schools included assessments of the various needs of children in poverty. Health care services are among the greatest needs and SBHCs are competing with other health programs to deliver such services. In New Jersey, for example, the state was ordered by the courts to reform its school finance system. As part of the state's response, the Department of Human Services contributed $6 million in state funds to establish or expand school health centers (First, Curcio, and Young, 1993). The SBHC at Jersey City's Snyder High was eligible for these funds but failed to carry out the requisite planning and community assessments (Interview, state health official, June 21, 1999). Nonetheless reforms in school funding offer opportunities for increased resources for many school health centers. To take advantage of these opportunities, SBHC advocates must be willing to lobby legislators and make their case in court if necessary.

MENTAL HEALTH SERVICES

School-based clinic providers claim that mental health counseling is the greatest unmet need among students (Allensworth et al., 1997). Estimates from the Department of Health and Human Services reveal that mental health problems affect approximately 20 percent of youth. As many as 12 percent of adolescents suffer from clinical depression, and according to the American Academy of Child and Adolescent Psychiatry, the rate of suicide among fifteen- to twenty-four-year-olds has tripled since 1960 (Kendell, 2000). Furthermore, significant numbers of American youth have serious drug abuse issues, and foremost among these substances is alcohol. Almost a third of high school seniors and a quarter of tenth graders reported heavy drinking (five or more drinks in a row within the past two weeks) in 1999 (*America's Children,* 2000). Depression and stress are other serious problems facing many youth, problems that have been exacerbated by the deteriorating and unsafe social conditions in which they live (Dryfoos, 1994; Weist, 2001).

"There's a tremendous need for more psychologists, especially after the violence in Littleton (Colorado), because students here have many of those problems too. Many of our students feel like there's no tomorrow," explained a Jersey City clinic official (Interview, May 19, 1999). Indeed, the report commissioned by Congress after those 1999 shootings at Columbine High School concluded that youth violence is an "epidemic" and occurs in conjunction with "drugs, guns, gangs, and sex, and teen-agers most likely to participate are low-income males" ("Report Details Youth Crime," 2001:5A). Thus, the importance of school-based health centers in offering mental health services cannot be overemphasized.

A variety of factors explain the insufficiency of mental health services for children and adolescents, including the lack of access to traditional sites where services are typically offered (such as community mental health centers), the fragmentation of services, the cost of mental health treatments and the difficulty in obtaining reimbursement from Medicaid and managed care, and the "stigma" associated with mental health problems. In addition, youth who exhibit depression or anxiety but demonstrate no obviously disruptive behaviors are difficult to identify (Bickham et al., 1998). While most secondary schools employ guidance counselors, they are in short supply and their emphasis is usually on academic matters such as course selection and college applications. Relatively few schools collaborate with community mental health workers to address more personal aspects of youth development. Even fewer schools employ psychologists or social workers (Dryfoos, 1994).

Although in some communities the provision of these services is controversial, mental health care is among the fastest-growing SBHC services. This reflects the "expanded school mental health services movement"—a shift in the provision of primary care from community mental health centers and private offices to schools (Weist, 2001: 101). Among those involved in this service delivery are counselors, psychologists, social workers, nurses, and psychiatrists. Obviously the SBHC can provide an effective coordinating center for the collaboration of these professionals' efforts (Flaherty et al., 1998).

Our 1998 national survey indicated that 79 percent of SBHCs are offering mental health counseling, and that this is by far the fastest-growing service in most clinics. The census of SBHCs in 1998-99 reported that clinic mental health services included crisis intervention (79 percent), case management (70 percent), comprehensive evaluation and treatment (69 percent), substance abuse (57 percent), and the assessment and treatment of learning problems (39 percent). A number of centers offered group counseling for peer support (59 percent), grief counseling (53 percent), classroom behavior modification (49 percent), substance abuse treatment (41 percent), and gang intervention (26 percent). With more and better mental health services, such counseling has become the leading reason for student visits to school clinics. Moreover studies have shown that the barriers experienced in traditional mental health settings—stigma, noncompliance, and inadequate access—are overcome in school-based settings (Schlitt et al., 2000).

Portland's Parkrose High School clinic expanded its services in 1994 to include a full-time mental health therapist. This service proved especially beneficial when the clinic became a neighborhood health center in 1997, serving not only students but their families and other adults. Adding a mental health professional enabled the center to give greater attention to issues of depression, eating disorders, family planning, drug abuse, and violence. According to a Parkrose school administrator:

> There's been an increased demand for mental health services. Students really want and need "someone to talk with," particularly students with special needs (i.e., disabled, physically abused, suicidal). We now even have a grieving group for those who have experienced the death or loss of a family member or friend. (Interview, June 26, 1998)

Mental health services in the form of a child psychiatrist were also begun at the East San Jose Elementary School clinic in Albuquerque in the mid-1990s. Health center personnel had perceived "great needs among the students, especially from the effects of domestic violence and substance abuse among parents" (Interviews, May 3-4, 1999). Moreover, the children had no access to counseling elsewhere due to a lack of transportation, no medical insurance, and cultural fear of people outside their neighborhood. A school official claimed that mental health services had enabled the clinic to "deal with the underlying problems" of many children, and to work with their parents (when willing) as well (Interview, May 4, 1999). In promoting such services in schools more generally, the RWJ Foundation recently allocated $3.4 million in grants to SBHCs to add or expand mental health or dental services (Making the Grade, 2001).

Yet we found that underfunded SBHCs in poorer communities with tremendous student needs often remain without mental health programs. Such programs are also rare where there are large numbers of traditional religious groups, indicating again the influence of opposition forces. On the other hand, more affluent suburban school health centers are more likely to offer counseling services than their rural or urban counterparts (see also Fothergill, 1998). Clinic budget cuts at Shanks High School (Quincy) and Snyder High School (Jersey City), meant that all services beyond primary care, including psychologists and social workers, were eliminated. "We have a real need for mental health services," stated a Snyder High School official. "We desperately need a psychologist who can deal preventively with violent-prone students and youth who desire to have children. Drugs, alcohol, deaths in the family, and students re-entering school after prison are all important yet neglected issues" (Interview, May 19, 1999).

DEALING WITH SEXUAL ORIENTATION

One service that almost all SBHCs have failed to offer is counseling, referral, and assistance with youth issues regarding sexual orientation and identity. Because of the serious consequences of living in a society that is often hostile toward homosexuality, bisexuality, and transgender status, youth that develop these identities often feel isolated, alienated, stressed, and depressed. Gay students, for example, are five times more likely than straight students to be the target of violence or abuse in school (National Gay and Lesbian Task Force, 2001). As a result, these youth are at high risk of such critical mental health problems as substance and alcohol abuse, and suicide. Although schools, especially those with SBHCs, are clearly in a position to offer care and help for these youth (e.g., counseling for youth as they struggle with accepting a homosexual identity, or dealing with the verbal and/or physical abuse they often face), the controversial nature of homosexuality has stymied most efforts. In fact, although some states such as Massachusetts have passed laws to protect gay and lesbian youth from harm in schools, many others such as North Carolina have passed legislation that prohibits school personnel from developing any programs that positively affirm a homosexual orientation.

Studies of school districts that have been able to offer services which prevent problems and offer assistance to gay and lesbian youth have documented that certain political strategies can be helpful in putting these services in place. First, the political environment is important. Large, diverse communities that are relatively affluent and located in progressive states are more likely to adopt school programs supportive of gay youth. Second, the political activity of gay citizens is also significant. School programs for gay and lesbian youth were greater in places where gays served in local public office and mobilized to influence school board elections. In Philadelphia, for example, where local and state officials were relatively supportive of gay rights, the city's Lesbian and Gay Task Force, a well-organized gay interest group, was the driving force in persuading schools to address sexual orientation issues (Button, Rienzo, and Wald, 1997).

In our survey, only 38 percent of SBHCs claimed to offer counseling for sexual orientation issues. Further analysis of the data indicated that relatively large progressive cities were most likely to offer such counseling. Our case study sites, however, experienced strong resistance to providing these services even though SBHC personnel recognized the need. According to a school official at Parkrose High (Portland):

> Our clinic does nothing on sexual orientation. Even a brief presentation related to this issue that was given to tenth graders resulted in several negative phone calls from parents. It's a very controversial issue here, but we have not dealt with it. There is a

need, however—a youth population that is not served and at high risk. (Interview, June 25, 1998)

SBHCs in Albuquerque are also beginning to confront issues involving gay youth. At East San Jose Elementary, clinic personnel discuss sexual orientation during the HIV/puberty program. In the high school health centers, some counseling is available to gay youth and two schools have developed gay-straight alliances. "The clinic advisory boards are discussing more services to support gay and lesbian students, but it's a very controversial topic," stated a SBHC official. "We [clinic personnel] want all students to understand antigay prejudice and its consequences" (Interview, May 3, 1999).

THE GENDER GAP

Adolescent girls are much more likely than boys to visit a school health center. Our national survey indicated that 59 percent of clinic users were female. The Advocates for Youth 1997 survey of SBHCs showed the same overall gender gap, with secondary schools reporting a higher average percentage of female users (61.6 percent) than primary schools (38.2 percent) (Fothergill, 1998). In addition, we found that teenage girls were attracted to the health centers largely by reproductive health services—that is, the greater the number of sexuality services offered, the larger the percentage of female users. Such visits by adolescent girls are important because if any serious discussions about sexual issues are to take place, they are most likely to be in the privacy of the school clinic where students know that conversations will be kept confidential (Emihovich and Herrington, 1997).

The gender gap in clinic use was a significant issue at every SBHC we visited. Studies of gender differences have indicated that females are more expressive and more likely than males to seek support when coping with stressful issues. Men's ways of coping tend to be more rational and stoic, and thus males are less likely to seek help in dealing with emotional issues (O'Leary and Helgeson, 1997; Thoits, 1991). Beyond differences in gender role socialization, teenage boys face other barriers that prevent them from visiting school health centers. Most clinics lack male doctors and other personnel with whom boys would feel more comfortable. Moreover, adolescent boys are sensitive to the negative reaction of peers to clinic users. In the words of a male student at Snyder High School (Jersey City):

> Some guys don't want to come to the health clinic; they think others will think they have a [sexually transmitted] disease, and *kids talk!* Also, there's no male doctor and some guys feel embarrassed about talking to or being examined by a female. (Interview, November 22, 1991)

Involving more boys in school health centers is a goal of virtually every clinic director. At Parkrose High School in Portland, clinic personnel conducted focus groups with males to investigate why boys do not visit the clinic more frequently. They learned that few boys knew about the SBHC and that males were more willing to visit a school health center than the community health department. As a result of this information, more publicity about the SBHC was generated, much of it coming through male teachers, counselors, and coaches (Interviews, June 26, 30, 1998).

At Snyder High in Jersey City, clinic staff encouraged male athletes and student leaders to support the clinic with the knowledge that such peer role models are influential among students. Females who visited the health center for reproductive services were strongly encouraged to bring along their boyfriends, and support groups established for troubled males proved to be helpful and popular (Interviews, May 19, 1999). Albuquerque's East San Jose clinic recruited male medical students and residents from the University of New Mexico and found this useful in attracting boys to the health center (Interview, April 30, 1992). In Quincy, the SBHC developed an adult male mentoring program to help students, especially boys. Men of Action, a black male service organization, was particularly instrumental in mentoring black youths, focusing on ways to resolve conflicts, to improve academic performance, and to seek advice and assistance with health and sexual issues through the school clinic (Interview, December 10, 1998).

In Virginia Beach, where there are no SBHCs, health professionals established a peer-mentoring program in two secondary schools with large numbers of at-risk students. In a thirteen-week program that focused on communication skills, decision making, healthy relationships, sexuality issues, suicide, and conflict resolution, 150 teen mentors were trained to provide accurate information and referrals for their peers.

With an emphasis on male mentors for troubled boys, this program gained the support of eleven local health and social service agencies that were also available for student referrals. Special T-shirts identified the peer mentors within their schools. The program proved so successful that plans were under way to expand it to other schools and to involve the NAACP Youth Council for greater outreach (Interview, May 29, 1998).

NEGLECT OF LATINOS

In 1997 the poverty rate among Hispanic youth was more than one in three (36 percent), almost 2.5 times the rate for non-Hispanic white youth (Rodgers, 2000). In addition, since 1994 the birthrate for Latino teenagers has been higher than that of other minority groups, including black teens (Curtin and Martin, 2000). Similarly, between 1991 and 1997 most adolescents, except for Hispanics, reported substantial declines in risk behaviors, such as weapon carrying, fighting, suicidal thoughts, and sexual intercourse. During the same period all teen groups including Latinos, reported increases in the use of marijuana, cocaine, and tobacco (Lindberg et al., 2000).

Although Hispanic children and adolescents participate in more high-risk behaviors than other racial or ethnic groups, they are least likely to be medically insured and to receive basic health care (Lindberg et al., 2000), including school-based health services. Our SBHC survey indicated that the larger the Latino school enrollment, the fewer the number of clinic services and hours of operation, and the smaller the student enrollment in and use of the health center. In a study of health services for youth, including SBHCs, in four major cities (New York, Baltimore, Philadelphia, and Washington, DC), it was reported that Hispanic youth have limited access to health care services (Acosta, Shafer, and Weist, 1999). The study found a lack of culturally sensitive health programs for Latinos, with language being the greatest barrier. Hispanic youth were also reluctant to seek services for cultural reasons, including the stigmas attached to Western medical approaches and the practice of keeping personal issues within the family.

Although SBHCs have focused on meeting the health needs of poor youth, Latino students have not benefitted to nearly the same extent as non-Hispanic whites and African Americans. Beyond the cultural explanations, there are several important political reasons for this condition. Unlike African Americans, the other sizable minority served by clinics, Hispanics are not politically well organized nor do they participate politically at high rates. Hispanics are a very diverse ethnic population made up of Mexican-Americans, Puerto Ricans, Cubans, and others from various countries in Central and South America. Each of these groups has somewhat distinct needs and goals, and are therefore difficult to mobilize politically as a cohesive Latino minority. In addition, difficulty with the English language, the presence of a sizable number of noncitizens, and lack of understanding of U.S. politics create formidable barriers for many Hispanics (McClain and Stewart, 1999). As a result, the percentage of adult Latinos who reportedly were registered (35 percent) and voted (27 percent) in the 1996 U.S. presidential election was among the lowest of any minority in the country (U.S. Bureau of the Census, 1998), a trend that has been apparent for several decades. Low levels of participation have translated into the election of relatively few Hispanics to local school boards and other city and state offices (McClain and Stewart, 1999).

Due to cultural barriers and lack of political clout, the growing health care needs of Latino youth have been overlooked by many SBHCs. A number of suggestions have been made for rectifying this omission and improving school health services for such youth (Acosta, Shafer, and Weist, 1999; Interviews, Albuquerque, May 3-5, 1999). First and perhaps most important, provide clinic and referral agency staffs with cultural education, including knowledge of the Spanish language. Second, create culturally sensitive programs that deal with the barriers often confronting Hispanic youth. Third, provide greater SBHC outreach to Latino students and their parents, both in and out of school. It is important to improve youth and parental access to basic information about school-based health care including enrollment procedures, services offered, confidentiality, and parent and student rights. Fourth, recruit Latino staff for the clinic. They will attract greater numbers of Hispanic youth while often serving as minority mentors and role models. Finally, work to gain the support of local and state political leaders, especially Latinos and other minorities, by making them aware of the significant health care needs of Hispanic children and adolescents.

UNDERUTILIZED RESOURCES

Business

School reforms, such as health centers, are most likely to survive and grow when they are actively supported by a broad cross section of community groups. Parents, educators, and health professionals clearly play a central role, but potentially business leaders are also a key element in the civic capacity for health and educational improvement (Orr, 1996; Stone, 1998). In most communities businesses are a dominant force in local politics not only because of their economic resources but also due to their civic associations and social status (Kweit and Kweit, 1999). In the words of Clarence Stone, "business has a long history of being highly valued as 'symbols of civic legitimacy'" (1998:255), and business involvement in local issues is considered highly important by public officials and community leaders.

Despite the widespread belief that linkages with politically and economically powerful groups can help to sustain SBHCs, few such relationships with businesses have been developed. Results from our national survey showed that business leaders were ranked very low by clinic directors in terms of the level of SBHC support provided by various community groups. Forty-three percent claimed no support from local businesses, and 18 percent perceived a low level of assistance. Many clinic personnel believed that businesses would not value relationships with school health centers because of the controversial nature of some services, the lack of awareness of the role played by clinics, and the general perception that students received health services elsewhere (Juszczak, Moody, and Vega-Matos, 1998). As a result, relatively few attempts have been made to develop meaningful partnerships between SBHCs and the business community.

The potential for forging relationships with business is great in many communities, and given the limited resources of many school clinics, the assistance of business can be extremely helpful. In attempting to develop relationships with the business community, clinic personnel might consider several approaches (Juszczak, Moody, and Vega-Matos, 1998). First, stress the role of SBHCs in education as well as health, and focus on the linkage between the two in promoting the development of healthy, skilled, educated, and productive citizens. Students, in turn, will ultimately contribute to the business community as employees, consumers, and as members of society in general. This approach appeals to the direct stake business leaders have in the quality of the labor pool and in the desire for economic growth and development.

Second, many businesses have a sense of civic responsibility and adopt an attitude of support for various community organizations as a matter of promoting good public relations. As a result, in recent decades there has been a growth in the willingness of businesses to assist schools and other organizations in fund-raising, provision of materials, and sharing of specialized staff resources (Orr, 1996). SBHCs can appeal to this sense of civic obligation by focusing on the health needs of children. Many business leaders are concerned about youth in the community in terms of sexuality issues, violence, drug abuse, problems in the home, and family life (Juszczak, Moody, and Vega-Matos, 1998). Educating the business community about the roles played by school health centers in meeting these youth needs is necessary in order to begin developing a supportive relationship.

Finally, SBHCs can construct a range of relationships with businesses depending on clinic needs and what businesses are able and willing to provide. Direct financial support may not be possible or desirable, especially at first. Nonetheless business participation may involve serving on boards and committees (especially the clinic's community advisory board), in-kind charitable contributions, joint education or training, collaborative projects, direct services, joint research efforts, and contractual arrangements. If some of these joint efforts prove successful, and further understanding and mutual trust are developed, businesses and SBHCs may forge long-term partnerships in which direct funding is possible. Such partnerships, however, need to be perceived as beneficial to both parties (Juszczak, Moody, and Vega-Matos, 1998). Given the status of the business community, once school health centers have gained the support of business leaders, other community organizations may follow the lead and become more willing to lend assistance.

Universities

University-based personnel and related resources have played a key role in developing school health programs and school reforms in general. The missions of scholarship (which involves generating grant monies, conducting research, and publishing scientific articles) and of teaching provide the basis for strong support. One way that university departments institutionalize their involvement is through establishing formal relationships with specific schools or school districts. These sites can be maintained as laboratories for testing programs and structural changes, for training preprofessional students, and for providing in-service education and ongoing consultation for school staffs (Dryfoos, 1994).

A significant factor in university involvement is the decision by the administration to commit to community-based projects. The SBHC at the East San Jose Elementary School (Albuquerque) has benefitted greatly from the involvement of the University of New Mexico, which is solidly committed to community outreach, especially to the medically underserved. The Department of Pediatrics started the clinic and has maintained its presence as strong supporters. The department's medical residents and students staff the SBHC, which has become a prime choice to fulfill the community project work that the medical school requires for graduation. The clinic work has been "well received by the medical students, the community, and the kids with needs. In addition, the medical residents (who make a two-year commitment) could follow kids over time, which has been very good for the residents" (Interview, medical school official, May 5, 1999). The university has been able to secure grant funding that provides for an SBHC coordinator for several school sites including East San Jose. This coordinator is a key position in maintaining financial and community support. More recently, the University's psychiatric department has begun to provide mental health services for the students and their families. The SBHC staff feels secure in its future due to the clear understanding that UNM's support is assured (Interviews, clinic staff, May 3-5, 1999).

Foundations

Foundations have often been "influential agents of change" in school reform (Orr, 1996:329). In New York, Chicago, Baltimore, and other cities local nonprofit foundations played significant roles in systemic reform. National foundations such as the Robert Wood Johnson, Carnegie, Ford, Kellogg, MacArthur, Pew, Annie E. Casey, and Grant have been instrumental in creating model education and health programs. They have initiated major multistate interventions and funded the research required to measure effects (Dryfoos, 1994). While often overlooked in the development of innovative programs, foundations control large amounts of resources, view themselves as agents of change, and are bound solely by the mission of the organization (Orr, 1996).

Foundations were crucial to the initiation of the first school-based health clinics. By the mid-1970s the first SBHCs attracted the attention of the Robert Wood Johnson Foundation, which funded model school health programs, including a SBHC in Posen-Robbins, Illinois. In the 1980s RWJ launched major funding ($12 million) for SBHC start-up projects and expanded this initiative in the 1990s. RWJ also organized Making the Grade, a project in ten states to develop district wide, comprehensive school health programs. Other foundations contributed as well. Ford and Carnegie Foundations funded the Support Center for School-Based Health Services whereby a national network of professionals was developed to foster the growing demand for SBHCs. This national communication system proved to be an important resource in the diffusion of school health centers (Sharp, 1997).

In 1987, Jersey City was one of nineteen sites nationwide to be awarded a $600,000 RWJ grant to establish a SBHC. The initial allocation of $200,000 covered start-up expenses for the Snyder High School Health Center, and the balance enabled the clinic to meet basic costs over the first four years (Leir, 1987). With no state monies available and a limited tax base, Jersey City would not have been able to develop the school clinic without foundation funding. Once foundation support ended, however, SBHC funding proved to be much less stable.

By the 1990s local and regional foundations became increasingly interested in supporting this innovative approach to health care for youth. In 1994, the Graustein Foundation pledged $2 million for SBHCs in four Connecticut cities. A year later the Kellogg Foundation gave $4 million in support of school health centers in Detroit, and in 1996 the Duke Endowment announced $3 million to fund clinics in North and South Carolina schools (Making the Grade, 1998). Thus private foundations have often been an important but relatively unexplored and untapped source of monetary and other resources for SBHCs.

Churches and Faith-Based Organizations

Religious groups often have a "strong interest in the ethical and moral development of young people" (Dryfoos, 1998:262). Communities of faith are committed to the general good of the community and are trusted institutions. Moreover, church members include people who are experienced in volunteering, providing monetary resources, and serving as youth advocates. Many church leaders have developed "bully pulpits" from which they influence the thinking of their parishioners, including the importance of helping youth to overcome social, economic, racial, and health barriers (Dryfoos, 1998; Juszczak, Moody, and Vega-Matos, 1998).

Some social scientists have argued that neighborhood-based service reforms are rarely successful without incorporating a spiritual approach to serving others. Such an approach provides a sense of dedication and understanding that is rarely found in more secular programs. It may also produce a more determined political commitment. As social scientist Glenn Loury has observed, "Successful efforts at reconstruction in ghetto communities invariably reveal a religious institution, or set of devout believers, at the center of the effort" (as quoted in Schorr, 1997:16).

In African-American communities, in particular, the roots of the church run deep enough to make it the focus of political and other organized activities. Black clergy continue to provide major political leaders (Wald, 1997). In Quincy, the Ministerial Alliance, composed of mostly African-American ministers, was a strong and important advocate for the Shanks SBHC. Furthermore, a leading black minister chaired the clinic's community advisory board, helped to plan the health center, and used church services along with his weekly local radio program to inform the public of the need for a high school clinic (Interviews, April 8, 1992). According to a school board member, "Ministers have been very supportive of the Shanks clinic. That's the way to sell something here . . . through the churches" (Interview, December 11, 1998).

Although connections between school health centers and religious organizations are possible and often useful to both partners, it is important to understand issues of potential contention. More traditional religious groups have often been the chief *opponents* of SBHCs, particularly to reproductive health services and to the diminished role of parents in the process of health care provision. In addition, some faith communities may be supportive solely in a self-serving attempt to attract people to their particular religious order.

Similarly, relatively few school clinics have any supportive connections with church groups. Our national survey indicated that SBHC directors perceived religious organizations as very low in the level of support for, and very high in opposition to, school health centers. Of the 65 percent of SBHCs with an active community advisory board, only a third reported having a representative of a religious group serving on their board.

Yet school health clinics and faith-based organizations overlap in interests and responsibilities, although they may focus on different issues (Juszczak, Moody, and Vega-Matos, 1998). Many religious communities have a long history of providing various social services to children and families. Developing connections with religious organizations could increase youth and family access to health services as well as create greater advocacy for shared issues involving SBHCs. As in the case of foundations and local businesses, faith communities tend to be a largely untapped source of assistance. President George W. Bush's recent emphasis on increased federal funding for faith-based organizations may provide the incentive necessary to secure such support.

POLITICAL ADVOCATES FOR YOUTH

Unlike most citizens in our society, children and teens, particularly those in need, are not able to politically advocate on their own behalf. Even for those who do speak out for youth, such as parents, teachers, and health and social service providers, there is often no clear consensus as to the causes or remedies for youth at risk. Although many liberals see growing child poverty as the basic issue, conservatives claim that the chief problem lies in parental irresponsibility, divorce, and unmarried motherhood. Which government programs, if any, are helpful is also a matter of intense debate (Skocpol, 2000).

In contrast to youth, the elderly are extremely well-organized politically and vote at higher rates than any other age group. As a result, government programs for older Americans are numerous and well funded, particularly Social Security and Medicare, the major programs benefitting the aging. With limited public budgets, youth have been shortchanged as seniors have reaped vast government benefits. Largely due to public programs, poverty among the aging has plummeted in recent decades. At the same time the rate of poverty among children and teenagers has increased dramatically (Rodgers, 2000).

Amid the debate over government programs for youth in need, school health centers are gaining support as a public intervention that is targeted and involves limited spending. What SBHCs lack is strong and consistent advocates, a problem shared with many programs for youth. Students served by such health clinics are among the most ardent supporters, but their voices are rarely heard beyond the school walls. It is important that students, particularly those in high school, lobby in political arenas such as school boards and public agencies where their testimonials may have a significant impact.

At Snyder High School in Jersey City, adolescents proved to be strong proponents of the health center. Their high rate of clinic usage was an endorsement in itself. Beyond this, some teens were outspoken advocates of the center, both in school and in the community. While these were not organized efforts, the comments of youth about the usefulness and economic advantage of the clinic in meeting their health needs were persuasive (Interviews, May 19, 1999).

Other advocates of children's school health services, including parents, educators, and health professionals, need to work to persuade politicians that SBHCs are cost-effective ways to provide primary care for underserved youth. The focus of these efforts is increasingly necessary at the state level where health care is typically high on the agenda, and where SBHCs are congruent with the goals of health care reform (Lear, 1996). As we have indicated, states are now the focal point for funding and new programs that reach children and adolescents in need.

ACCOUNTABILITY

The ultimate ability to sustain SBHCs will depend greatly on establishing evidence of success. The people who support (financially and otherwise) these clinics will call for proof that they "work" in ways that truly meet the needs of the youth served and the goals of funding organizations. As a result, it is crucial for clinics to be able to document that they effectively contribute to youth's educational and personal well-being.

Critics of SBHCs are quick to push for indicators of outcomes to prove that clinics are not successful and therefore a waste of money. Even advocates often fear outcomes accountability. Many communities have expectations for the effects of school clinics on their children that greatly exceed possibilities, and funders sometimes demand immediate evidence of success. Moreover, measuring important outcomes, such as effects on teen pregnancy, are difficult to gauge, and significant factors that contribute to youth problems are often outside the control of SBHCs. Thus although SBHCs may be able to partially contribute to a decrease in some of the most important causes of morbidity and mortality in youth, it is imperative to focus on realistic expectations and measures.

Several strategies promote the process of identifying and managing accountability studies. First, the right outcome measures on which to focus must be selected. In the words of social analyst Lisbeth Schorr, "The initial challenge is to get everybody who has a stake, including skeptics, to agree on a set of outcomes considered important, achievable, and measurable" (Schorr, 1997:122). Once there is agreement on outcomes, a clear identification of the measures to be used for indicating such outputs is required. In this regard, SBHCs should utilize their resources wisely. For example, in the funding request there needs to be monies devoted to outcome measurement. In addition, the SBHCs should procure the involvement of experts available to them, such as university professors who do research as part of their responsibilities, to assist in this endeavor. Furthermore, technical assistance is usually available from state and national agencies, such as state departments of health, the Center for Health and Health Care in Schools, and the National Assembly of School-Based Health Centers.

Second, outcome measures need to be easy to understand and compelling, not only to experts and decision makers, but also to parents and the community in general. For example, process measures, such as counting the numbers of youth that the clinic serves, provide evidence of activity that the clinic is "successful" in reaching youth. Dollar costs per user, one legitimate indicator of cost effectiveness, is also readily obtainable data. Both funders and program people need and want these types of data. However, in the policy evaluation process, it is a mistake to focus only on indicators that are persuasive to supporters. In addition, the distinction between outcomes and processes often becomes confused, and the emphasis on what actually happens to children as a result of the SBHC is lost (Making the Grade, 1997). For example, indicators of the numbers of youth visiting the clinic is not nearly as important as measures of the impact of the health center on prevention of morbidity or increasing school attendance.

Quality outcome measures are still unrefined; there is a dearth of long-term studies measuring the breadth of clinic impact. Moreover, even at their best, outcomes-based measures may not capture the full effects of clinic interventions. For example, we do not yet know what the impacts of clinics are on adult health and education status for those who had SBHC support during their school years. Yet these types of effects are the most important indicators of what the program is really accomplishing (Schorr, 1997). Investigating long-term success requires a lengthy period to carry out as well as a significant investment of funds. To assist in this effort, we strongly recommend the utilization of both quantitative and qualitative data measures over time that will more fully represent a clinic's impact. Again, this is an expensive and time-consuming project, but one critically tied to the sustainability and growth of SBHCs.

Portland's Multnomah County Health Department has been a strong force from the outset in the development of assessments of their SBHCs. The Parkrose High School clinic directly benefitted from important data collection processes—youth health needs, support of parents to establish the clinic, and clinic usage—that served to document its effectiveness. For instance, a survey in 1994 showed that "parents in general were highly supportive of SBHCs' involvement in teen pregnancy prevention efforts" and proved helpful in enabling Parkrose to expand its efforts in this area (Interview, public health official, June 30, 1998). Clinic personnel also collected and utilized persuasive qualitative data appropriately. As an example, clinic advocates cited the testimony of a Parkrose parent who praised the SBHC because his daughter was able to access birth control that "allowed her to finish high school" (Interview, public health official, June 30, 1998). Multnomah County truly has been a determined pioneer in establishing sophisticated techniques to assess SBHCs.

Another important component of assessment is making sure that clinic results are publicized and presented to leaders with political clout at both the local and state levels. The Gadsden County Health Department was successful in this endeavor in the initial years of Shanks High School's SBHC. Douglas Kirby, a nationally renowned expert on evaluation of school-based health programs, was commissioned to head a study that included the Shanks clinic. When the results of this and other studies were published, the newspaper headline proclaimed "Neighborhood Clinic Praised; Teenage Pregnancies Reduced by Approximately 75 Percent," and cited that this testimony had been provided to the Florida House Health Care Committee as well. Soon after this report, several state legislators and other political leaders toured the clinic and gave it high praise (Harper, 1989:1).

DEALING WITH THE RACE ISSUE

Most school districts, even those in largely minority urban areas, downplay the importance of race and ethnicity. White Americans assume that serious racial issues in schools have been resolved, and that blacks and Latinos are relatively content with the educational system. Even many racial minorities, having witnessed the incorporation of blacks and Latinos into education politics through election to school boards and appointment to administrative posts, believe that political power translates into improved education. These optimistic views buttress a positive vision of quality education for all. Recent studies, however, have portrayed grave disappointment in local education by African Americans and Latinos who have assumed power (Browning, Marshall, and Tabb, 1997; Henig et al., 1999; Rich, 1996).

Race (and ethnicity to a lesser extent) continues to be a major influence in education policy, including the politics of school health centers. Explicit racial distrust and conflict are evident, particularly in inner cities where minorities and SBHCs are concentrated. A history of struggles over school desegregation, community control of schools, funding of minority-dominated schools, and other racial issues have made it difficult for minorities and whites to cooperate and sustain relationships. As a result, local multiracial political coalitions are difficult to develop and maintain. Race also establishes barriers to white business leaders, politicians, parents, and other community groups that might otherwise participate in school reform. White business and other community elites fear becoming enmeshed in racial issues, while African-American and Latino school and city officials often face criticism from minority parents for working with white leaders (Henig et al., 1999). Even beyond the confines of the community, race and ethnicity influence education politics. State legislatures and courts, for example, often make important decisions affecting school and health care funding and regulations, and race is clearly a factor in a number of these actions.

With substantial economic and political resources controlled by whites, the critical task is to develop intergroup cooperation and organizations that include both minority and white leaders. Since funding and broad community support are crucial issues for SBHCs, many of which serve primarily minority youth, policymakers often need to bridge racial divisions. Several strategies serve to facilitate reaching this goal.

First, it is important initially to focus on limited but achievable goals. As mentioned previously, demonstrating that school-based centers can help reduce student absenteeism or school dropout rates, for example, is the kind of small success that encourages participation and support across the community. SBHCs are often able to produce limited, measurable gains in a cost-effective manner, thus appealing to white business and other leaders. Moreover, early success, particularly with minority students, suggests that school health center interventions may also be helpful in reducing more serious morbidities such as teen pregnancy, STDs, crime, and school violence. These are communitywide goals shared by minority and white citizens alike.

Second, minority leaders must attempt to build confidence and trust with white individuals and groups that have shown that they are reliable allies, willing to work with African-American and Latino communities (Henig et al., 1999). This may not include a white superintendent or mayor who is in a position of power but is not necessarily connected in any way to the minority community. White leaders new to the community, for example, are typically unknown outsiders with no developed networks of relationships. Our study has demonstrated that minority school board members, administrators, and other city officials have the power and legitimacy to develop individual intergroup connections that are so important to breaking down racial distrust. Including a range of racially diverse individuals on the

SBHC advisory board is one way to promote improved race relations. Such relationships are also the first step toward forging permanent biracial coalitions that provide the communitywide support necessary for SBHC growth and longevity. In addition, minority leaders would do well to encourage the establishment of school health centers in predominantly white schools as well, thus showing mutual support for SBHCs and demonstrating to whites how useful clinics can be for all students.

"MODEL" SBHC REFORM

In her large-scale analysis of interventions that actually work to increase the success of high-risk youth, Lisbeth Schorr (1997) describes four features of such reform efforts by schools. First, schools link with services that are available in the community. Second, the school complex (buildings, fields, playgrounds) becomes accessible to residents in the neighborhood. Third, forming partnerships with other organizations in the community is important. Last, successful school reform involves families. School-based health centers, carefully established and sustained, can credibly fulfill the criteria requisite to successful school reform efforts. We will discuss the SBHC in Parkrose High School (Portland) again to illustrate this model for all of these aspects of reform.

Parkrose's SBHC is a subsidiary of the Multnomah County Health Department. Thus it provides all the medical care services traditionally available to citizens through public health but is more accessible as a neighborhood clinic. Although housed in the school, the administration of the SBHC is maintained by the county health department, and the clinic remains open after traditional school hours, several evenings each week, and in the summer. In addition, it provides services to adults in the area as well as youth, including youth that have dropped out of school. Teachers are kept well informed of clinic services for referral and, because of its expanded hours, they know that students do not have to leave class (and therefore miss academic work) to attend to their health needs. Linking to available health and social services succeeds only when "a dependable and appropriate set of services and supports are in place for teachers to mobilize" (Schorr, 1997:286). In addition, schools, by opening their facilities to the neighborhood, have "many parents and other residents feeling connected to these schools in a way they never were before" (Schorr, 1997:287). Thus Schorr's major directives with respect to the first and second types of school reform efforts are evident at the Parkrose clinic.

Schorr also found that effective reform involves the partnership of schools with "informal helping networks, including church and social ties, family support services, youth development programs, mentoring, recreational opportunities, and strong bonds among adults" (287) so that schools are not solely responsible in the effort. This third aspect of reform has also clearly developed at Parkrose. The "Caring Community" concept with its mission "to build strong schools and keep kids in school" has been supported at the state, county, and school district levels and by city and county leaders and elected officials (Interview, school administrator, June 24, 1998). At the county level, this has translated into a "tremendous commitment by county commissioners to the SBHC. They supply the funding for the clinics. They are proud to have adopted, as their mission, the importance of providing health care to citizens, especially for poor kids" (Interview, public health official, June 30, 1998).

Further evidence of this outreach to the community in partnership emerged in response to the need for funding to expand the school's services, including the SBHC. As described previously, approval of a bond issue required three votes, but by the last one the community had gone through a visioning process and worked out a plan that placed several key community services in the school facility. These included a performing arts center, computer education center, police department outpost, as well as the expanded SBHC as an arm of the health department. Furthermore, the SBHC works closely with the community's family resource center, the local Lutheran church's Family Works program, the school booster club, and the SBHC can count on the support of the Oregon Medical Association, local pediatricians, family practice physicians, and psychiatrists (Interviews, public health official, June 30, 1998; school health official, June 24, 1998).

Finally, Schorr noted that successful school reform efforts involve families as valued partners because "all children learn best when parents and teachers share a similar vision, when there is a 'sense of constancy'" (1997:288). This, too, has been carefully developed by the school and county at Parkrose through the SBHC. Each school and community representative interviewed about the Parkrose clinic described parents as "highly supportive" of the clinic. From the outset, parents' opinions and needs were surveyed, and services were shaped based on their responses. "There are very few complaints" and "once parents find out what we do, they are supportive because they view it as another help to their child" (Interviews, school board member, June 24, 1998; school clinic official, June 24, 1998).

POLITICS AS THE KEY

Proponents of school health centers have become more aware of the political issues involved in developing and maintaining these unique programs of health care for youth. From gaining and sustaining funding to offering controversial services such as reproductive and mental health care, many SBHCs have confronted difficult political issues. What school clinic advocates have learned is that politics matters a great deal in the success or failure of SBHCs (Rienzo, Button, and Wald, 2000).

Enlisting the cooperation and support of both the inner and outer core of personnel in the school and community is essential. Students, teachers, parents, school administrators, as well as key leaders and organizations in the larger community, need to be made aware that SBHCs provide competent, accessible, and trustworthy care that meets the needs of students. Once confidence and trust in school health centers are developed, clinics are eventually able to expand services to include reproductive health care (Zeanah et al., 1996).

Building civic capacity, or the mobilization of various stakeholders in support of a community or school reform, calls for "exercising political leadership and mastering political skills" (Henig et al., 1999:9). Civic capacity involves seeing an issue as a community problem that calls for a collective response. It also means participation or involvement so as to contribute to the reform (Stone, 1998). Developing civic capacity in school systems and communities where large numbers of students come from families who live below the poverty line is a major challenge. For most SBHCs, the health care needs of youth are great and the delivery of resources is difficult. Nevertheless there is no route to reform *around* politics—even a reform as modest as an SBHC. Indeed, because of the limits on local governments and resources, it is imperative to build coalitions to exercise influence at the state and even national levels. These larger jurisdictions are crucial in providing the greater financial and other support necessary for school health centers to survive.

The importance of developing civic capacity is emphasized by a state department of health official in New Mexico, a person with significant experience in the development of SBHCs:

> The recipe for success of school health centers is school and community support, with little political conflict. The school board, superintendent, nurses, teachers, and other school personnel need to support it, along with the community. SBHC collaboration with providers is important as well, as is having a strong clinic advocate or two. And sufficient funding is necessary, which means developing positive relations with local and state sources. (Interview, May 5, 1999)

School-based health centers are increasingly seen as a very useful component of health care for youth. Most clinics are relatively small in size, and they are still limited in number. Thus they are no substitute for Medicaid, managed care, or private health insurance. Yet SBHCs do complement these traditional health care approaches in very important ways. Indeed, school clinics have distinctive advantages in reaching and serving youth, particularly those that are disadvantaged. Most SBHCs provide active outreach, encourage repeat visits, and offer an accessible, friendly place where children and adolescents may talk about their anxieties or high-risk behaviors that often underlie their health problems. They provide health education, mental health counseling, and reproductive services that are rarely readily available to youth. In addition, school health centers aid working parents who find it difficult to take time off for sick children. They have also proved to be a relatively inexpensive way to offer health care to underserved youth (Marone , Kilbreth, and Langwell, 2001). In terms of effectiveness, SBHCs have helped to reduce school absenteeism and dropouts, pregnancies, STDs, drug abuse, and other morbidities among some of the most troubled youth.

Recently the U.S. Surgeon General David Satcher, upon releasing a major public health report, proclaimed that "Schools must be the great equalizer in assuring that all children have a basic understanding of essential sexual health matters" (Connolly, 2001:A16). It appears that SBHCs are a health policy whose time has come. They have moved beyond the policy innovation stage and have gained increased acceptance across the states. Politically, school health centers are perceived as a health care solution for youth that is not too costly and does not require major reform efforts. SBHCs have arrived on the political scene at the very time schools face pressing problems of youth violence, substance abuse, and sexuality issues.

Most Americans are supportive of programs that improve the family and the lives of children, yet are locally controlled and not associated with "big government". Although school health centers alone are no panacea, they do offer hope, especially for poor and minority youth with the highest morbidities. Increasingly state legislators and other politicians of both major parties are viewing school clinics as a health care reform that works. With a growing national concern for education and health care, the time is politically ripe for school-based health clinics.

References

Chapter 1

Allensworth, Diane, Elaine Lawson, Lois Nicholson, and James Wyche (Eds.). 1997. *Schools and Health: Our Nation's Investment*. Washington, DC: National Academy Press.

American Academy of Pediatrics. 1993. *School Health: Policy and Practice*. Elk Grove Village, IL: Author.

Bar-Cohen, Annette, Betty Lia-Hoagberg, and Laura Edwards. 1990. "First Family Planning Visit in School-Based Clinics," *Journal of School Health* 60(8): 418-422.

Crosby, Richard A., and Janet St. Lawrence. 2000. "Adolescents' Use of School-Based Health Clinics for Reproductive Health Services: Data from the National Longitudinal Study of Adolescent Health," *Journal of School Health* 70(1): 22-27.

Dryfoos, Joy G. 1985. "School-Based Health Clinics: A New Approach to Preventing Adolescent Pregnancy?" *Family Planning Perspectives* 17(2): 71-75.

Dryfoos, Joy G. 1991. "School-Based Social and Health Services for At-Risk Students," *Urban Education* 26(1):118-137.

Dryfoos, Joy G. 1994. *Full-Service Schools: A Revolution in Health and Social Services for Children, Youth and Families*. San Francisco: Jossey-Bass Publishers.

Dryfoos, Joy G. 1998. *Safe Passage: Making It Through Adolescence in a Risky Society*. New York: Oxford University Press.

Durlak, Joseph A. 1995. *School-Based Prevention Programs for Children and Adolescents*. Thousand Oaks, CA: Sage Publications.

Eng, T.R., and W.T. Butler (Eds.). 1997. *The Hidden Epidemic: Confronting Sexually Transmitted Diseases*. Washington, DC: National Academy Press.

Fothergill, Kate. 1998. *Update 1997: School-Based Health Centers*. Washington, DC: Advocates for Youth.

General Accounting Office. 1994. *Health Care Reform: School-Based Health Centers Can Promote Access to Care*. Washington, DC: General Accounting Office.

Hyche-Williams, H. Jean, and Cynthia Waszak. 1990. *School-Based Clinics: Update 1990*. Washington, DC: Center for Population Options.

Isaacs, Stephen L., and James R. Knickman (Eds.). 1999. *To Improve Health and Health Care, 1999: The Robert Wood Johnson Foundation Anthology*. San Francisco: Jossey Bass.

Jaynes, Gerald David, and Robin M. Williams Jr. (Eds.). 1989. *A Common Destiny: Blacks and American Society*. Washington, DC: National Academy Press.

Kirby, Douglas, Cynthia Waszak, and Julie Ziegler. 1991. "Six School-Based Clinics: Their Reproductive Health Services and Impact on Sexual Behavior," *Family Planning Perspectives* 23(1): 6-16.

Kort, M. 1984. "The Delivery of Primary Health Care in American Public Schools, 1890-1980," *Journal of School Health* 54(11): 453-457.

Making the Grade. 1991. "HIV in Teens Challenges Schools, Health Centers," *Access to Comprehensive School-Based Health Services for Children and Youth* (spring).

Making the Grade. 1998. "Exploring the Evolution of School-Based Health Centers," *Access to Comprehensive School-Based Health Services for Children and Youth* (winter). Washington, DC: Author.

McCord, M.T., J.D. Klein, J.M. Foy, and K. Fothergill. 1993. "School-Based Clinic Use and School Performance," *Journal of Adolescent Health* 14: 96-97.

Means, R.K. 1975. *Historical Perspectives on School Health*. Thorofare, NJ: Charles B. Slack.

Office of Technology Assessment, Congress of the United States. 1991. *Adolescent Health*. Washington, DC: U.S. Government Printing Office.

Peterson, Paul. 1981. *City Limits*. Chicago, IL: University of Chicago Press.

Rienzo, Barbara A. 1994. "Factors in the Successful Establishment of School-Based Clinics," *The Clearing House* 67(6): 356-362.

Rienzo, Barbara A., and James W. Button. 1993. "The Politics of School-Based Clinics: A Community-Level Analysis," *Journal of School Health* 63(6): 266-272.

Rosenau, Pauline V. (Ed.). 1994. *Health Care Reform in the Nineties*. Thousand Oaks, CA: Sage.

Schuster, Mark A., Robert M. Bell, Sandra H. Berry, and David E. Kanouse. 1998. "Impact of a High School Condom Availability Program on Sexual Attitudes and Behaviors," *Family Planning Perspectives* 30(2): 67-72, 88.

Sharp, Elaine B. (Ed.). 1999. *Culture Wars and Local Politics*. Lawrence, KS: University Press of Kansas.

Stone, Clarence N. (Ed.). 1998. *Changing Urban Education*. Lawrence, KS: University Press of Kansas.

Stone, Clarence, Kathryn Doherty, Cheryl Jones, and Timothy Ross. 1998. "Schools and Disadvantaged Neighborhoods: The Community Development Challenge." Unpublished paper, 45 pp.

U.S. Public Health Service. 1991. *Healthy People 2000: National Health Promotion and Disease Prevention Objectives*. Washington, DC: U.S. Government Printing Office.

Velsor-Friedrich, B. 1995. "Schools and Health, Part II: School-Based Clinics," *Journal of Pediatric Nursing* 10(1):62-63.

Weathersby, Ann M., Marie L. Lobo, and Deborah Williamson. 1995. "Parent and Student Preferences for Services in a School-Based Clinic," *Journal of School Health* 65(1): 14-17.

Wirt, Frederick M., and Michael W. Kirst. 1989. *Schools in Conflict: The Politics of Education*. Berkeley, CA: McCutchan Publishing.

Chapter 2

Allensworth, Diane, Elaine Lawson, Lois Nicholson, and James Wyche (Eds.). 1997. *Schools and Health: Our Nation's Investment.* Washington, DC: National Academy Press.

Annual Progress Report: Snyder High School. 1991. Jersey City, NJ: Snyder High School School-Based Health Center.

Averett, Nancy. 1998. "School Nurses Give Help," *Herald and News,* August 3: 1, 4A.

Bickham, Nicole L., Josefina Pizarro, Beth S. Warner, Bernice Rosenthal, and Mark D. Weist. 1998. "Family Involvement in Expanded School Mental Health," *Journal of School Health* 68(10):425-428.

Birk, Ed. 1986. "Seesaw Battle Goes on over School Clinic in Gadsden," *Tallahassee Democrat,* September 17: 2B.

Bobo, Lawrence, and Ryan A. Smith. 1994. "Antipoverty Policy, Affirmative Action, and Racial Attitudes." In Danziger, Sheldon H., Gary D. Sandefur, and Daniel H. Weinberg (Eds.), *Confronting Poverty: Prescriptions for Change* (pp. 365-395). New York: Russell Sage Foundation.

Button, James. 1989. *Blacks and Social Change: Impact of the Civil Rights Movement in Southern Communities.* Princeton, NJ: Princeton University Press.

Center for Human Services Policy and Administration. 1989. *Shanks Health Center Evaluation Final Report: Third Year of Program Operation.* Tallahassee, FL: Center for Human Services Policy and Administration.

"Clinic Concept Is Praiseworthy." 1985. *Gadsden News,* August 15.

Clolery, Paul. 1987. "School Sex Ed Clinics Stirring up Passions," *The Jersey Journal,* May 8: 1, 16.

Colburn, David R., and Lance deHaven-Smith. 1999. *Government in the Sunshine State.* Gainesville, FL: University Press of Florida.

Danielson, Michael, and Jennifer Hochshield. 1998. "Changing Urban Education: Lessons, Cautions, Prospects." In Stone, Clarence N. (Ed.), *Changing Urban Education* (pp. 277-295). Lawrence, KS: University Press of Kansas.

Davis, Marc. 1986a. "Beach Refuses to Fund Teen Pregnancy Study," *The Virginian-Pilot,* May 9: D1, 4.

Davis, Marc. 1986b. "Parents Attack Pregnancy-Prevention Plan," *The Virginian-Pilot,* April 30: D1.

Dietrich, Matthew. 1988. "Teen Clinic Quietly Opens," *The Hudson Dispatch,* March 24: 1,16.

Doherty, Katheryn M., Cheryl L. Jones, and Clarence N. Stone. 1998. "Building Coalitions, Building Communities: The Challenge of Collaboration." Working paper 23 for National Center for the Revitalization of Central Cities, University of New Orleans.

Dooley, Pat. 1998. "Youths Are Urged to Delay Sex," *The Virginian-Pilot,* May 29: B1, 7.

Dryfoos, Joy G. 1994. *Full-Service Schools: A Revolution in Health and Social Services for Children, Youth and Families.* San Francisco: Jossey-Bass Publishers.

Dryfoos, Joy G. 1998. "School-Based Health Centers in the Context of School Reform," *Journal of School Health* 68(10): 404-408.

Dryfoos, Joy, and John Santelli. 1992. "Involving Parents in Their Adolescents' Health: A Role for School Clinics," *Journal of Adolescent Health* 13: 259-260.

DuPont-Smith, Alice. 1991. "Clinic Is Moved Back to Campus After Three Years Across the Street," *Gadsden County Times,* January 10: 3.

DuPont-Smith, Alice. 1993. "Two Schools Will Get Full Service Health Centers," *Gadsden County Times,* January 28: 2.

Dye, Thomas R. 2000. *Politics in States and Communities.* Upper Saddle River, NJ: Prentice Hall.

Editorial. 1998. "Sex Ed Wrong Time to Backpedal," *The Virginian-Pilot,* May 10: J4.

Emihovich, Catherine, and Carolyn D. Herrington. 1997. *Sex, Kids, and Politics: Health Services in Schools.* New York: Teachers College Press.

Fiedler, Tom. 1986. "Forum to Discuss Quincy Clinic Also Served a Political Purpose," *Tallahassee Democrat,* May 22:11A.

Final Report: A Compilation of Service Center Activities. 1995. Quincy, FL: James A. Shanks High School Student and Family Service Center.

Flaherty, Lois T., Ellen G. Farrsion, Robyn Waxman, Patricia F. Uris, Susan G. Keys, Marcia Glass-Siegel, and Mark D. Weist. 1998. "Optimizing the Roles of Mental Health Professionals," *Journal of School Health* 68(10): 420-424.

Fothergill, Kate. 1998. *Update 1997: School-Based Health Centers.* Washington, DC: Advocates for Youth.

Gittell, Marilyn. 1980. *Limits to Citizen Participation.* Beverly Hills, CA: Sage.

Hacker, Karen, and Genie L. Wessel. 1998. "School-Based Health Centers and School Nurses: Cementing the Collaboration," *Journal of School Health* 68(10): 409-413.

Harper, Jack. 1989. "Neighborhood Clinic Praised: Teenage Pregnancies Reduced by Approximately 75 percent," *Gadsden County Times,* October 19: 1.

Harper, Jack. 1990. "Reduced Pregnancies Here May Lead to New Bill," *Gadsden County Times,* March 29: 2.

Hunter, James Davison. 1991. *Culture Wars: The Struggle to Define America.* New York: Basic Books.

Johnston, Rhonda. 1998. "School-Based Health Centers in the Western Region of the United States and Their Long-Term Financial Viability," Fort Collins, CO: Colorado State University. Unpublished doctoral dissertation.

King, Ledyard. 1998. "Sex Education in Schools," *The Virginian-Pilot,* February 13: A1.

Kirby, Douglas, Cynthia S. Waszak, and Julie Zielgler. 1989. *An Assessment of Six School-Based Clinics: Services, Impact and Potential.* Washington, DC: Center for Population Options.

Kweit, Robert W., and Mary Grisez Kweit. 1999. *People and Politics in Urban America*. New York: Garland Publishing.

Laws, Page. 1986. "Sex Education Remains One of the Most Controversial Issues in Our Classrooms," *The Virginian-Pilot,* February 23: J1-2.

Leir, Ronald. 1986a. "School Clinics May Dispense Contraceptives," *The Jersey Journal,* December 12: B1.

Leir, Ronald. 1986b. "School's Contraception Unlikely," *The Jersey Journal,* December 15: B1.

Leir, Ronald. 1987. "Snyder to Get Pilot Clinic," *The Jersey Journal,* May 28: 1, 12.

Leir, Ronald. 1989. "Snyder High Clinic Now Accepted by Students," *The Jersey Journal,* November 7:14.

Lindley, Lisa L., Belinda M. Reininger, and Ruth P. Saunders. 2001. "Support for School-Based Reproductive Health Services Among South Carolina Voters," *Journal of School Health* 71(2): 66-72.

Making the Grade. 1993. "Education and Health: Bridging the Barriers," *Access to Comprehensive School-Based Services for Adolescents* (winter/spring).

Making the Grade. 1998. *School-Based Health Centers in Virginia 1997-1998*. Washington, DC: Author.

Making the Grade. 1999. "SBHCs Are Making the Grade with Teachers." *Access to Comprehensive School-Based Services for Adolescents* (pp. 1-2, 4). Washington, DC: Author.

Making the Grade. 2000. "Why Are Some SBHCs Closing?" *Access to Comprehensive School-Based Health Services for Children and Youth* (spring): 1-4.

"Many Eligible Families Lack Health Benefits." 2000. *Gainesville Sun:* August 10: 6A.

Mayfield, Marjorie. 1986. "Lake Taylor Chosen for Health Clinic," *The Virginian-Pilot,* November 14.

Nieves, Evelyn. 1997. "Showing Teen-Age Girls the Virtue of Abstinence," *The New York Times,* August 7.

"Poor Kids May Never See Funds." 2000. *Gainesville Sun,* July 11: 1, 5A.

Pulley, Brett. 1997. "Parity in Schools," *The New York Times,* May 15.

Reed, Douglas S. 1994. "The People v. The Court: School Finance Reform and the New Jersey Supreme Court," *Cornell Journal of Law and Public Policy* 4: 137-198.

Reed, Douglas S. 1998. "Twenty-Five Years After *Rodriguez:* School Finance Litigation and the Impact of the New Judicial Federalism," *Law and Society* 32(1): 175-219.

Regan, Elizabeth. 1986. "Prevention: Teen Pregnancy Battle Begins," *The Virginian-Pilot,* February 21: A1-2.

Regan, Elizabeth. 1987. "School Sex Clinic Given Funds," *The Ledger Star,* February 19.

Rich, Wilbur C. 1996. *Black Mayors and School Politics: The Failure of Reform in Detroit, Gary, and Newark*. New York: Garland Publishing.

Rienzo, Barbara A., and James W. Button. 1993. "The Politics of School-Based Clinics: A Community-Level Analysis," *Journal of School Health* 63(6): 266-272.

Rienzo, Barbara A., James W. Button, and Kenneth D. Wald. 2000. "Politics and the Success of School-Based Health Centers," *Journal of School Health* 70(8): 331-337.

Rodgers, Harrell R. Jr. 1979. *Poverty Amid Plenty: A Political and Economic Analysis.* Reading, MA: Addison-Wesley Publishing Company.

Rozell, Mark J., and Clyde Wilcox. 1996. *Second Coming: The New Christian Right in Virginia Politics.* Baltimore, MD: The Johns Hopkins University Press.

Santelli, John, Mary Vernon, Richard Lowry, Jenny Osorio, Martha DuShaw, Mary Sue Lancaster, Ngoc Pham, Elisa Song, Elizabeth Ginn, and Lloyd J. Kolbe. 1998. "Managed Care, School Health Programs, and Adolescent Health Services: Opportunities for Health Promotion," *Journal of School Health* 68(1): 434-440.

School Division Facts. 1997. Virginia Beach, VA: Virginia Beach City Public Schools.

"School Equity in New Jersey." 1996. *The New York Times,* May 27.

Stone, Clarence N. (Ed.). 1998. *Changing Urban Education.* Lawrence, KS: University Press of Kansas.

Sussman, Paul. 1987. "Beach Parents Battle Sex Education," *The Virginian-Pilot,* November 18: D1, 3.

U.S. Bureau of the Census. 1990. *Census of Population: General Social and Economic Characteristics. Final Report.* Washington, DC: U.S. Government Printing Office.

Washington, Susan. 1986. "School Clinic Spurs Controversy," *Gadsden County Times,* January 16: 1.

Weathersby, Ann M., Marie L. Lobo, and Deborah Williamson. 1995. "Parent and Student Preferences for Services in a School-Based Clinic," *Journal of School Health* 65(1):14-17.

Wilcox, Clyde. 1996. *Onward Christian Soldiers?: The Religious Right in American Politics.* Boulder, CO: Westview Press.

Wooten, Gregory. 1985a. "Parents Object to Clinic," *Gadsden County Times,* October 17: 2.

Wooten, Gregory. 1985b. "School Clinic Plan Gets Partial," *Gadsden County Times,* September 26: 1.

Chapter 3

Allensworth, Diane, Elaine Lawson, Lois Nicholson, and James Wyche (Eds.). 1997. *Schools and Health: Our Nation's Investment.* Washington, DC: National Academy Press.

American Medical Association Council on Scientific Affairs. 1989. "Providing Medical Services Through School-Based Programs," *Journal of the American Medical Association* 261(23): 1939-1942.

Brostrom, Molly B., and Ian T. Hill. 1993. *Opportunities for Enhancing Preventive and Primary Care Through School-Based Health Centers: Three States' Title V Program Experiences.* Washington, DC: Association of Maternal and Child Health Programs.

Dryfoos, Joy G. 1991. "School-Based Social and Health Services for At-Risk Students," *Urban Education* 26(1): 118-137.

Dryfoos, Joy G. 1994. "Medical Clinics in Junior High School: Changing the Model to Meet Demands," *Journal of Adolescent Health* 15: 549-557.

Dye, Thomas R. 2000. *Politics in States and Communities.* Upper Saddle River, NJ: Prentice Hall.

Elders, M. Joycelyn. 1993. "Schools and Health: A Natural Partnership," *Journal of School Health* 63(7): 312-315.

Emihovich, Catherine, and Carolyn D. Herrington. 1997. *Sex, Kids, and Politics: Health Services in Schools.* New York: Teachers College Press.

Fothergill, Kate. 1998. *Update 1997: School-Based Health Centers.* Washington, DC: Advocates for Youth.

Fox, Harriette B., Lori B. Wicks, and Debra J. Lipson. 1992. "Improving Access to Comprehensive Health Care Through School-Based Programs." Report to U.S. Department of Health and Human Services, Washington, DC.

Graber, Doris A. 1984. *Media Power in Politics.* Washington, DC: CQ Press.

Hacker, Karen, and Genie L. Wessel. 1998. "School-Based Health Centers and School Nurses: Cementing the Collaboration," *Journal of School Health* 68(10): 409-413.

Howley, Nora. 2000. "School Centers Help Often-Overlooked Youths," *The Washington Post,* July 9: B5.

Johnston, Rhonda. 1998. School-Based Health Centers in the Western Region of the United States and Their Long-Term Financial Viability. Fort Collins, CO: Colorado State University. Unpublished doctoral dissertation.

Juszczak, Linda, Jacob K. Moody, and Carolos Vega-Matos. 1998. "Business and Faith: Key Community Partnerships for School-Based Health Centers," *Journal of School Health* 68(10): 429-433.

Kaniss, Phyllis. 1995. *The Media and the Mayor's Race: The Failure of Urban Political Reporting.* Bloomington, IN: Indiana University Press.

Klein, J.D., S.A. Starnes, and M. Lotelchuck. 1990. *Comprehensive Adolescent Health Services in the United States.* Chapel Hill, NC: The Cecil G. Sheps Clinic for Health Services Research.

Kweit, Robert W., and Mary Grisez Kweit. 1999. *People and Politics in Urban America.* New York: Garland Publishing.

Lear, Julia Graham. 1996. "Health Care Goes to School: An Untidy Strategy to Improve the Well-Being of School-Age Children." In Irwin Garfinkel, Jennifer L. Hochschild, and Sara S. McLanahan (Eds.), *Social Policies for Children.* Washington, DC: The Brookings Institution.

Making the Grade. 1995. "States Lead the Way for School-Based Health Centers," *Access to Comprehensive School-Based Health Services for Children and Youth* (winter): 1-2.

Making the Grade. 1996. "Louisiana's School-Based Health Centers Secure $2.6 Million Annual Appropriation," *Access to Comprehensive School-Based Health Services for Children and Youth* (summer): 1-3.

Making the Grade. 1998. "Exploring the Evolution of School-Based Health Centers," *Access to Comprehensive School-Based Health Services for Children and Youth (*winter): 1-4.

Making the Grade. 1999. "SBHC Associations Proving There Is Strength in Numbers," *Access to Comprehensive School-Based Health Services for Children and Youth* (summer): 1-3.

Making the Grade. 2000a. "Fact Sheets—New Mexico." Available online at <www.gwu.edu/~mtg/temp/NM.htm> (June 3, 2000).

Making the Grade. 2000b. "State Coalitions." Available online at <www.gwu.edu/~mtg>.

Miller, Christopher. 1987. "APS Board Votes to Keep Clinics," *The Albuquerque Journal,* August 6: A1-2.

Moore, Charles. 1987. "Intense Debate Continues Over School Health Clinics," *The Albuquerque Journal,* July 7: B2.

Orr, Marion. 1996. "Urban Politics and School Reform: The Case of Baltimore," *Urban Affairs Review* 31(3): 314-345.

Pacheco, Mario, Wayne Powell, Catherine Cole, Norton Kalishman, Robert Benon, and Arthur Kaufman. 1991. "School-Based Clinics: The Politics of Change," *Journal of School Health* 61(2): 92-94.

Rienzo Barbara A. 1994. "Factors in the Successful Establishment of School-Based Clinics," *The Clearing House* 67(6): 356-362.

Rienzo, Barbara A., and James W. Button. 1993. "The Politics of School-Based Clinics: A Community-Level Analysis," *Journal of School Health* 63(6): 266-272.

Rienzo, Barbara A., James W. Button, and Kenneth D. Wald. 2000. "The Politics of School-Based Health Centers," *Journal of School Health* 70(8): 331-337.

Rindini, Steven P. 1998. *Health and Sexuality Education in Schools: The Process of Social Change.* Westport, CT: Bergin and Garvey.

Santelli, John, Miriam Alexander, Mychelle Farmer, Pat Papa, Tonya Johnson, Bernice Rosenthal, and Dana Hotra. 1992. "Bringing Parents into School Clinics: Parent Attitudes Toward School Clinics and Contraception," *Journal of Adolescent Health* 13: 269-274.

Santelli, John, Anthony Kouzis, and Susan Newcomer. 1996. "Student Attitudes Toward School-Based Health Centers," *Journal of Adolescent Health* 18: 349-356.

Santelli, John, Madlyn Morreale, Alyssa Wigton, and Holly Grason. 1996. "School Health Centers and Primary Care for Adolescents: A Review of the Literature," *Journal of Adolescent Health* 18: 357-366.

Schlitt, John, John Santelli, Clare Brindis, Robert Nystrom, Jonathan Klein, and M.D. Seibou. 2000. *Creating Access to Care: School-Based Health Center Census 1998-99.* Washington, DC: National Assembly on School-Based Health Care.

Stadell, Cynthia. 1989. "Parkrose Teen Health Clinic," Portland, OR: Parkrose School District Public Information Office.

Steineger, Melissa. 1989. "Possible Clinic at Parkrose High School Raises Concern," *The Oregonian,* June 27: B2.

Stern, Henry. 1998. "New Parkrose High School Fulfills Promise," *The Oregonian,* January 22: 1.

Stone, Clarence (Ed.). 1998. *Changing Urban Education.* Lawrence, KS: University Press of Kansas.

University of New Mexico Health Sciences Center. 1998. "Demographics of East San Jose School," *At the Health Center: East San Jose.* Albuquerque, NM: Author.

U.S. Bureau of the Census. Online 1990 Census Fact Finder: <http://factfinder. census.gov/java_prod/dads.ui.fac.CommunityFactsPage>.

Walter, Heather J., Roger D. Vaughan, Bruce Armstrong, Roberta Y. Krakoff, Lorraine Tiezzsi, and James F. McCarthy. 1995. "School-Based Health Care for Urban Minority Junior High School Students," *Archives of Pediatric Adolescent Medicine* 149: 1221-1225.

Weathersby, Ann M., Marie L. Lobo, and Deborah Williamson. 1995. "Parent and Student Preferences for Services in a School-Based Clinic," *Journal of School Health* 65(1): 14-17.

Wirt, Frederick M., and Michael W. Kirst. 1989. *Schools in Conflict.* Berkeley, CA: McCutchan Publishing Corporation.

Zook, Ronald (Parkrose School district superintendent). 1989. Letter to Parkrose High School parents, September 7.

Chapter 4

Allensworth, Diane, Elaine Lawson, Lois Nicholson, and James Wyche (Eds.). 1997. *Schools and Health: Our Nation's Investment.* Washington, DC: National Academy Press.

American Academy of Pediatrics. 1993. *School Health: Policy and Practice.* Elk Grove Village, IL: Author.

Annual Progress Report. 1991. Jersey City, NJ: Snyder High School.

Auerbach, Stuart. 1996. "Lost Opportunities?" *Washington Post,* January 16: 8.

Button, James W., Barbara A. Rienzo, and Kenneth D. Wald. 1997. *Private Lives, Public Conflicts: Battles over Gay Rights in American Communities.* Washington, DC: Congressional Quarterly Press.

Center for Health and Health Care in Schools. 2000. "School-Based Health Centers: Results from a 50-State Survey School Year 1999-2000." Available online: <http://www. healthinschools.org/sbhcs/survey2000.htm>.

Centers for Disease Control and Prevention. 1999. "Trends in HIV-Related Sexual Risk Behaviors Among High School Students—Selected U.S. Cities, 1991-1997," *Journal of School Health* 69(7): 255-257.

Crosby, Richard A., and Janet St. Lawrence. 2000. "Adolescents' Use of School-Based Clinics for Reproductive Health Services: Data from the National Longitudinal Study of Adolescent Health," *Journal of School Health* 70(1): 22-27.

Dryfoos, Joy G. 1985. "School-Based Health Clinics: A New Approach to Preventing Adolescent Pregnancy?" *Family Planning Perspectives* 17(2): 70-75.

Dryfoos, Joy G. 1994. *Full-Service Schools: A Revolution in Health and Social Services for Children, Youth and Families.* San Francisco: Jossey-Bass Publishers.

Dryfoos, Joy, and John Santelli. 1992. "Involving Parents in Their Adolescents' Health: A Role for School Clinics," *Journal of Adolescent Health* 13: 259-260.

Emihovich, Catherine, and Carolyn D. Herrington. 1997. *Sex, Kids, and Politics: Health Services in Schools.* New York: Teachers College Press.

Fothergill, Kate. 1998. *Update 1997: School-Based Health Centers.* Washington, DC: Advocates for Youth.

Hunter, James Davison. 1991. *Culture Wars: The Struggle to Define America.* New York: Basic Books.

Hyche-Williams, H. Jean, and Cynthia Waszak. 1990. *School-Based Clinics: Update 1990.* Washington, DC: Center for Population Options.

Jones, Elise F., Jacqueline Darroch Forrest, Noreen Goldman, Stanley K. Henshaw, Richard Lincoln, Jeannie I. Rossoff, Charles F. Westoff, and Deirdre Wulf. 1985. "Teenage Pregnancy in Developed Countries: Determinants and Policy Implications," *Family Planning Perspectives* 17(2): 53-63.

Kann, Laura, Steven A. Kinchen, Barbara I. Williams, James G. Ross, Richard Lowry, Jo Anne Grunbaum, Lloyd J. Kolbe, and State and Local YRBSS Coordinators. 2000. "Youth Risk Behavior Surveillance—United States, 1999," *Journal of School Health* 70(7): 271-285.

Kirby, Douglas, Michael D. Resnick, Blake Downes, Thel Kocher, Paul Gunderson, Sandra Pothoff, Daniel Zelterman, and Robert William Blum. 1993. "The Effects of School-Based Clinics in St. Paul on School-Wide Birthrates," *Family Planning Perspectives* 25(1): 12-16.

Leir, Ronald. 1986. "School Clinics May Dispense Contraceptives," *The Jersey Journal,* December 12: B1.

Marone, James A., Elizabeth H. Kilbreth, and Kathryn M. Langwell. 2001. "Back to School: A Health Care Strategy for Youth," *Health Affairs* 20(1): 122-136.

Meier, Kenneth J. 1994. *The Politics of Sin: Drugs, Alcohol, and Public Policy.* Armonk, NY: M.E. Sharp.

Meier, Kenneth J., and Joseph Stewart. 1991. *The Politics of Hispanic Education.* Albany, NY: SUNY Press.

Meier, Kenneth J., Joseph Stewart, and Robert E. England. 1989. *Race, Class, and Education: The Politics of Second-Generation Discrimination.* Madison, WI: University of Wisconsin Press.

Missionaries to the Unborn. 2000. "Stop Public School Abortion Clinics in California." Available online: <http://www.mttu.com/>.

Moen, Matthew C. 1992. *The Transformation of the Christian Right*. Tuscaloosa, AL: The University of Alabama Press.

Mooney, Christopher Z. (Ed.). 2001. *The Public Clash of Private Values: The Politics of Morality Policy*. New York: Chatham House Publishers.

The National Campaign to Prevent Teen Pregnancy. 2001. "Facts and Stats: United States Pregnancy Rates for Teens, 15-19." Available online: <www.teenpregnancy.org/fedprate. htm>.

Pacheco, Mario, Wayne Powell, Catherine Cole, Norton Kalishman, Robert Benon, and Arthur Kaufman. 1991. "School-Based Clinics: The Politics of Change," *Journal of School Health* 61(2): 92-94.

Rienzo, Barbara A., and James W. Button. 1993. "The Politics of School-Based Clinics: A Community-Level Analysis," *Journal of School Health* 63(6): 266-272.

Santelli, John, Miriam Alexander, Mychelle Farmer, Pat Papa, Tonya Johnson, Bernice Rosenthal, and Dana Hotra. 1992. "Bringing Parents into School Clinics: Parent Attitudes Toward School Clinics and Contraception," *Journal of Adolescent Health* 13: 269-274.

Schlitt, John, John Santelli, Clare Brindis, Robert Nystrom, Jonathan Klein, and M.D. Seibou. 2000. *Creating Access to Care: School-Based Health Center Census 1998-99*. Washington, DC: National Assembly on School-Based Health Care.

Seligmann, Jean. 1987. "A Challenge to School Clinics," *Newsweek,* August 10: 54.

Sharp, Elaine B. (Ed.). 1999. *Culture Wars and Local Politics*. Lawrence, KS: University Press of Kansas.

Tatalovich, Raymond, and Byron W. Daynes (Eds.). 1998. *Moral Controversies in American Politics: Cases in Social Regulatory Policy*. Armonk, NY: M.E. Sharp.

Wald, Kenneth D. 1992. *Religion and Politics in the United States*. Washington, DC: CQ Press.

Wald, Kenneth D. 1997. *Religion and Politics in the United States*. Washington, DC: CQ Press.

Wald, Kenneth D., James W. Button, and Barbara A. Rienzo. 2001. "Morality Politics vs. Political Economy: The Case of School-Based Health Centers," *Social Science Quarterly* 82(2): 221-233.

Waszak, Cynthia, and Shara Neidell. 1991. *School-Based and School-Linked Clinics*. Washington, DC: Center for Population Options.

Wilcox, 1996. *Onward Christian Soldiers?: The Religious Right in American Politics*. Boulder, CO: WestviewPress.

Wilson, Thomas C. 1995. "Urbanism and Unconventionality: The Case of Sexual Behavior," *Social Science Quarterly* 76(2): 346-363.

Wooten, Gregory. 1985. "School Clinic Plan Gets Partial," *Gadsden County Times,* September 26: 1.

Zeanah, Paula D., Edward V. Morse, Patricia M. Simon, Mary Stock, Jo Lynn Pratt, and Sylvia Sterne. 1996. "Community Reactions to Reproductive Health Care at Three School-Based Clinics in Louisiana," *Journal of School Health* 66(7): 237-241.

Chapter 5

Acosta, Olga M., Michael E. Shafer, and Mark D. Weist. 1999. *Meeting the Needs of Latino Youth Through School-Based Programs.* Paper presented at the Annual Conference of the American School Health Association, Kansas City, MO, October 28.

Allensworth, Diane, Elaine Lawson, Lois Nicholson, and James Wyche (Eds.). 1997. *Schools and Health: Our Nation's Investment.* Washington, DC: National Academy Press.

America's Children: Key National Indicators of Well-Being, 2000. Federal Interagency Forum on Child and Family Statistics. <http//www.childstats.gov/ac2000/highlight.asp>.

Bickham, Nicole L, Josefina Pizarro, Beth S. Warner, Bernice Rosenthal, and Mark D. Weist.1998. "Family Involvement in Expanded School Mental Health," *Journal of School Health* 68(10): 425-428.

Bland, Karina. 2001. "School Health Clinics Fight for Lives," *Arizona Republic,* March 12.

Browning, Rufus P., Dale Rogers Marshall, and David H. Tabb (Eds.). 1997. *Racial Politics in American Cities.* New York: Longman.

Button, James W., Barbara A. Rienzo, and Kenneth D. Wald. 1997. *Private Lives, Public Conflicts: Battles Over Gay Rights in American Communities.* Washington, DC: Congressional Quarterly Press.

Center for Health and Health Care in Schools. 2001. *School-Based Health Centers: Results from a 50-State Survey.* Washington, DC: Author.

Connolly, Ceci. 2001. "Surgeon General Urges Inclusive Sex Education." *Washington Post,* June 29: A1, A16.

Curtin, Sally C., and Joyce A. Martin. 2000. *Births: Preliminary Data for 1999.* Hyattsville, MD: U.S. Department of Health and Human Services.

Dryfoos, Joy G. 1994. *Full-Service Schools: A Revolution in Health and Social Services for Children, Youth and Families.* San Francisco: Jossey-Bass Publishers.

Dryfoos, Joy G. 1998. *Safe Passage: Making It Through Adolescence in a Risky Society.* New York: Oxford University Press.

Emihovich, Catherine, and Carolyn D. Herrington. 1997. *Sex, Kids, and Politics: Health Services in Schools.* New York: Teachers College Press.

First, Patricia F., Joan L. Curcio, and Dalton L. Young. 1993. "State Full-Service School Initiatives: New Notions of Policy Development," *Politics of Education Association Yearbook* 8(5-6): 63-73.

Flaherty, Lois T., Ellen G. Farrsion, Robyn Waxman, Patricia F. Uris, Susan G. Keys, Marcia Glass-Siegel, and Mark D.Weist. 1998. "Optimizing the Roles of Mental Health Professionals," *Journal of School Health* 68(10): 420-424.

Fothergill, Kate.1998. *Update 1997: School-Based Health Centers*. Washington, DC: Advocates for Youth.

Greenblatt, Alan. 2000. "Lucky Strike," *Governing* (October): 42-45.

Harper, Jack. 1989. "Neighborhood Clinic Praised; Teenage Pregnancies Reduced by Approximately 75 Percent," *Gadsden Times,* October 19: 1.

Henig, Jeffrey R., Richard C. Hula, Marion Orr, and Desiree S. Pedescleaux. 1999. *The Color of School Reform: Race, Politics, and the Challenge of Urban Education*. Princeton, NJ: Princeton University Press.

Juszczak, Linda, Jacob K. Moody, and Carolos Vega-Matos. 1998. "Business and Faith: Key Partnerships for School-Based Health Centers," *Journal of School Health* 68(10): 429-433.

Kendell, Nicole. 2000. *Health Policy Tracking Service: School-Based Mental Health*. Washington, DC: National Conference of State Legislatures.

Koppelman, Jane, and Julia Graham Lear. 1998. "The New Child Health Insurance Expansions: How Will School-Based Health Centers Fit In?" *Journal of School Health* 68(1): 441-446.

Kweit, Robert W., and Mary Grisez Kweit. 1999. *People and Politics in Urban America*. New York: Garland Publishing.

Lear, Julia Graham. 1996. "Health Care Goes to School: An Untidy Strategy to Improve the Well-Being of School-Age Children." In Garfinkel, Irwin, Jennifer L. Hochschild, and Sara S. McLanahan (Eds.), *Social Policies for Children* (pp. 173-201). Washington, DC: The Brookings Institute.

Lear, Julia Graham. 2001. "Press Release: School-Based Health Centers Continue Strong Expansion Across the U.S., National Survey Finds," Washington, DC: The Center for Health and Health Care in Schools, March 1.

Lear, Julia Graham, Nancy Eichner, and Jane Koppelman. 1999. "The Growth of School-Based Health Centers and the Role of State Policies," *Archives of Pediatric and Adolescent Medicine* 153: 1177-1180.

Leir, Ronald. 1987. "Snyder to get Pilot Clinic," *Jersey City Journal,* May 28: 1, 12.

Lindberg, Laura D., Scott Boggess, Laura Porter, and Sean Williams. 2000. *Teen Risk-Taking: A Statistical Portrait*. Washington, DC: Urban Institute.

Making the Grade. 1997. "Taking Stock of School-Based Health Centers," *Access* (spring). Washington, DC: Author.

Making the Grade. 1998. "Exploring the Evolution of School-Based Health Centers," *Access* (winter). Washington, DC: Author.

Making the Grade. 2001. "Moving Forward: Making the Grade Becomes the Center for Health and Health Care in Schools," *Access* (winter). Washington, DC: Author.

Marone, James A., Elizabeth H. Kilbreth, and Kathryn M. Langwell. 2001. "Back to School: A Health Care Strategy for Youth," *Health Affairs* 20(1): 122-136.

McClain, Paula D., and Joseph Stewart Jr. 1999. *"Can We All Get Along?" Racial and Ethnic Minorities in American Politics*. Boulder, CO: Westview Press.

Meyer, Jack A., and Sharon Silow-Carroll. 2000. *Increasing Access: Building Working Solutions*. Washington, DC: Economic and Social Research Institute.

National Conference of State Legislatures, 2001. "Partisan Control of State Legislatures, 1938-2000." Available online: <http://www.nesl.org/programs/legman/elect/hstptyct.htm>.

National Gay and Lesbian Task Force. 2001. *Report*. Washington, DC: Author.

O'Leary, Ann, and Vicki S. Helgeson. 1997. "Psychosocial Factors and Women's Health: Integrating Mind, Heart, and Body." In Sheryle J. Gallant, Gwendolyn Puryear Keita, and Renee Royak-Schaler (Eds.), *Health Care for Women: Psychological, Social, and Behavioral Influences* (pp. 25-40). Washington, DC: American Psychological Association.

Orr, Marion. 1996. "Urban Politics and School Reform: The Case of Baltimore," *Urban Affairs Review* 31(3): 314-345.

Reed, Douglas S. 1998. "Twenty-Five Years after *Rodriguez:* School Finance Litigation and the Impact of the New Judicial Federalism," *Law and Society Review* 32(1): 175-219.

"Report Details Youth Crime." 2001. *Gainesville Sun,* January 18: 5A.

Rich, Wilbur C. 1996. *Black Mayors and School Politics: The Failure of Reform in Detroit, Gary, and Newark.* New York: Garland Publishing.

Rienzo, Barbara A., James W. Button, and Kenneth D. Wald. 2000. "Politics and the Success of School-Based Health Centers," *Journal of School Health* 70(8): 331-337.

Rodgers, Harrell R. Jr. 2000. *American Poverty in a New Era of Reform*. Armonk, NY: M.E. Sharpe.

Schlitt, J., J. Santelli, L. Juszczak, C. Brindis, R. Nystrom, J. Klein, D. Kaplan, and M.D. Seibou. 2000. *Creating Access to Care: School-Based Health Center Census 1998-1999*. Washington, DC: National Assembly on School-Based Health Care.

Schorr, Lisbeth B. 1997. *Common Purpose: Strengthening Families and Neighborhoods to Rebuild America*. New York: Doubleday.

Sengupta, Somini. 2001. "Health Agency Seeks to Close 27 Clinics," *New York Times,* May 15.

Sharp, Elaine B. 1997. "Money, Politics, and School Health Services: A New Look at State Policy Innovation." Unpublished paper.

Skocpol, Theda. 2000. *The Missing Middle: Working Families and The Future of American Social Policy*. New York: W.W. Norton and Co.

Stone, Clarence N. (Ed.). 1998. *Changing Urban Education*. Lawrence, KS: University Press of Kansas.

Thoits, P.A. 1991. "Gender Differences in Coping with Emotional Distress," in J. Eckenrode (Ed.), *The Social Context of Coping* (pp. 107-138). New York: Plenum.

U.S. Bureau of the Census. 1998. Voting and Registration in the Election of 1996. Washington, DC: U.S. Government Printing Office.

Wald, Kenneth D. 1997. *Religion and Politics in the United States*. Washington, DC: 1997.

Weist, Mark D. 2001. "Toward a Public Mental Health Promotion and Intervention System for Youth," *Journal of School Health* 71(3): 101-104.

Wirt, Frederick M., and Michael W. Wirt. 1989. *Schools in Conflict*. Berkeley, CA: McCutchan Publishing Corporation.

Zeanah, Paula D., Edward V. Morse, Patricia M. Simon, Mary Stock, Jo Lynn Pratt, and Sylvia Sterne. 1996. "Community Reactions to Reproductive Health Care at Three School-Based Clinics in Louisiana," *Journal of School Health* 66(7): 237-241.

Index

*For Product Safety Concerns and Information please contact
our EU representative GPSR@taylorandfrancis.com Taylor & Francis
Verlag GmbH, Kaufingerstraße 24, 80331 München, Germany*

T - #0136 - 270225 - C0 - 212/152/10 - PB - 9780789012722 - Gloss Lamination